Cancer Etiology, Diagnosis and Treatment

SQUAMOUS CELL CARCINOMA

Cancer Etiology, Diagnosis and Treatments

Additional books in this series can be found on Nova's website
under the Series tab.

Additional E-books in this series can be found on Nova's website
under the E-book tab.

Cancer Etiology, Diagnosis and Treatment

SQUAMOUS CELL CARCINOMA

DANIEL V. MORTENSEN
EDITOR

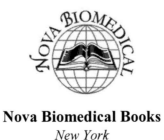

Nova Biomedical Books
New York

Copyright © 2011 by Nova Science Publishers, Inc.

For permission to use material from this book please contact us:
Telephone 631-231-7269; Fax 631-231-8175
Web Site: http://www.novapublishers.com

NOTICE TO THE READER

The Publisher has taken reasonable care in the preparation of this book, but makes no expressed or implied warranty of any kind and assumes no responsibility for any errors or omissions. No liability is assumed for incidental or consequential damages in connection with or arising out of information contained in this book. The Publisher shall not be liable for any special, consequential, or exemplary damages resulting, in whole or in part, from the readers' use of, or reliance upon, this material. Any parts of this book based on government reports are so indicated and copyright is claimed for those parts to the extent applicable to compilations of such works.

Independent verification should be sought for any data, advice or recommendations contained in this book. In addition, no responsibility is assumed by the publisher for any injury and/or damage to persons or property arising from any methods, products, instructions, ideas or otherwise contained in this publication.

This publication is designed to provide accurate and authoritative information with regard to the subject matter covered herein. It is sold with the clear understanding that the Publisher is not engaged in rendering legal or any other professional services. If legal or any other expert assistance is required, the services of a competent person should be sought. FROM A DECLARATION OF PARTICIPANTS JOINTLY ADOPTED BY A COMMITTEE OF THE AMERICAN BAR ASSOCIATION AND A COMMITTEE OF PUBLISHERS.

Additional color graphics may be available in the e-book version of this book.

Library of Congress Cataloging-in-Publication Data

Squamous cell carcinoma / editor, Daniel V. Mortensen.
   p. ; cm.
 Includes bibliographical references.
 ISBN 978-1-61209-929-3 (hardcover)
 1. Squamous cell carcinoma. I. Mortensen, Daniel V.
 [DNLM: 1. Carcinoma, Squamous Cell. QZ 365]
 RC280.S5S68 2011
 616.99'4--dc22
               2011005839

Published by Nova Science Publishers, Inc. † New York

CONTENTS

Preface   **ix**

Chapter 1   Squamous Cell Carcinoma Ontogeny: Part I   **1**
                 S Díaz Prado, V Medina Villaamil,G Aparicio Gallego,
                 R García Campelo and LM Anton Aparicio

Chapter 2   Squamous Cell Carcinoma Ontogeny: Part II   **37**
                 S Díaz Prado, G Aparicio Gallego, V Medina Villaamil,
                 R García Campelo and LM Anton Aparicio,

Chapter 3   Regulation of Cell Proliferation in Oral
                 Squamous Cell Carcinoma   **69**
                 Marcelo Donizetti Chaves, Mariza Akemi Matsumoto,
                 Patrícia Pinto Saraiva and Daniel Araki Ribeiro

Chapter 4   Squamous Cell Carcinoma Arising in Epidermal
                 Cyst and Human Papillomavirus Associated Cyst   **89**
                 Teresa Pusiol

Chapter 5   Epidermolysis Bullosa and
                 Squamous Cell Carcinoma   **107**
                 Minhee Kim, Lizbeth RA Intong
                 and Dedee F Murrell

Chapter 6   Dynamic Alteration of Nucleolin and AgNOR
                 Proteins in Oral Cancer Apoptotic Cells
                 by Ultraviolet Rays Irradiation   **123**
                 Shinji Kito, Shunji Shiiba, Masafumi Oda,

Tatsurou Tanaka, Yuji Seta, Nao Wakasugi-Sato,
Shinobu Matsumoto-Takeda, Izumi Yoshioka
and Yasuhiro Morimoto

Chapter 7   Squamous Cell Carcinoma of Tongue: Less Invasive
                   Surgical Approaches to Tongue Carcinomas   137
                   Masaaki Kodama, Amit Khanal, Manabu Habu,
                   Izumi Yoshioka, Takeshi Nishikawa, Hiroki Tsurushima,
                   Yusuke Yanagida, Shinji Kito, Tatsurou Tanaka,
                   Yasuhiro Morimoto and Kazuhiro Tominaga

Chapter 8   Oral Cuniculatum Carcinoma: Literature
                   Review   147
                   Yoann Pons

Chapter 9   Imaging of Squamous Cell Carcinoma   153
                   Lorenzo Faggioni, Emanuele Neri, Pietro Bemi,
                   Eugenia Picano, Francesca Pancrazi,Veronica Seccia,
                   Luca Muscatello,Stefano Sellari Franceschini
                   and Carlo Bartolozzi

Chapter 10   Emerging Non-Invasively Collected Genomic
                   and Proteomic Biomarkers for the Early Diagnosis of
                   Oral Squamous Cell Carcinoma (OSCC)   197
                   Joel A. Kooren, Nelson L. Rhodus
                   and Timothy J. Griffin

Chapter 11   Over Expression of P53 and P21 in Normal Oral
                   Mucosa Adjacent to Resected Squamous Cell
                   Carcinomas May Be an Evidence of Field
                   Cancerization   211
                   Reda F. Elgazzar, Aiman A. Ali, Ezzat Eldreeny
                   and Khalid Moustafa

Chapter 12   Laryngeal Squamous Cell Carcinoma: Treatment
                   Options and Outcomes   227
                   William M. Mendenhall, Russell W. Hinerman,
                   Robert J. Amdur, Mikhail Vaysberg
                   and John W. Werning

Contents

Index **247**

PREFACE

Squamous cell carcinoma (SCC) is a form of cancer of the carcinoma type that may occur in many different organs, including the skin, lips, mouth, esophagus, urinary bladder, prostate, lungs, vagina and cervix. This new book presents topical research in the study of the ontogeny of squamous cell carcinoma with a focus on the regulation of cell proliferation in oral squamous cell carcinoma. Also discussed is squamous cell carcinoma arising in epidermal cysts and human papillomavirus associated cysts and oral cuniculatum carcinoma

Chapter 1- Populations of cancer stem cells (CSCs) have been found and characterized in multiple malignancies as many cancers; however, this has not fully happened yet in human squamous cell carcinomas (SCC) of the lung, cervix and head & neck.

The field of stem cell biology is growing and will result in the steady identification of multi-potent, self-renewing, and proliferative progenitor's cell populations. These cells give rise to both transiently amplifying (TA) and terminally differentiated (TD) cells, which are important for tissue maintenance.

In leukemia, for example, it has been shown that partially committed cells, which are normally responsible for tissue maintenance after trauma may undergo transformation via mutations resulting in the selective expression of genes that accentuate and perpetuate these cells'self-renewal capabilities.

Bearing this in mind, it is valid to view stem cells as pro-tumorigenic. It has been proposed that the accumulation of oncogenic events may *lock* activated stem cells in a permanent aberrant state, which converts normal homeostatic stem cells into *cancer stem cells*. Because many developmental signaling pathways drive these cells into neoplasia, authors are required to understand, in some detail, their intricacies.

The observation that the earlier stage of human organ development to which a human tumor resembled was linked with worse survival rates suggested that abnormally-activated embryological cell signaling pathways are important in carcinogenesis. In order for an organism to develop, its cells need to be able to proliferate and to follow specific fates of cellular differentiation in a tightly controlled temporospatial manner, to ultimately ensemble and organize into functioning tissue and organs. Cell fate specification and complex gene regulatory networks (GRN) control development.

Cellular phenotypes are the result of patterns of gene expression. Intrinsic transcription factors released by cells in a timely manner provide the coordinates that delineate their individual fate. Extrinsic factors influence cells as groups through the process of differentiation. The integration of intrinsic and extrinsic cues is the decisive denominator, providing the coordinates of cell fate and differentiation. By understanding the interplay between these factors, we will hopefully dissect the processes leading to cell fate assignment.

As authors continue to understand, in detail, the repercussions of deregulation in key embryonic signaling pathways, the authors begin to dissect their intricate relationships with the stem cells and malignancy. Authors can explain how aberrations inflicted in many of the components of this complex homeostatic engine can lead to the formation of cancer stem cells with accumulated permanent mutations that allow them to re-populate their tumors rendering these lesions.

Research data from the last two decades suggests that there are four main signaling transduction pathways in the cell: Wnt, Hedgehog, Notch, and Bone morphogenic proteins. They are thought to act in parallel, to ultimately enhance specific genes that results in cell type-specific combinations of transcription factors responsible for cellular behavior, representing the basic machinery for determination of embryonic cell fate determination.

In this chapter, the authors explore the roles of the main developmental signaling pathways in organogenesis and maintenance, together with the issue of homeostatic stem cells within specific *niches* in the lung and maxillofacial tract. The aim, of course, is to ultimately integrate the knowledge of these mechanisms into tangible tools that can be eventually translated into novel therapies against the human cancers.

Chapter 2- Intermediary filaments, like cytokeratins, are essential intracellular components, underlying reflecting distinct cellular properties and differentiation stages in epithelial organs. The proteins of the cytokeratin family are epithelium specific expressed as low and high-molecular weight, acid and basic polypeptides. In general, CK expression patterns are highly-conserved. Cytokeratins (CKs) are the intermediate filament proteins of the epithelium cells which have become important markers of normal and abnormal cell differentiations. The keratin expression pattern in oral stratified epithelium is related to the cellular differentiation level: the normal pattern shows the keratin pair K5/14 in the stratum basale whereas K1/10 and k4/13, respectively, are the two pairs associated with differentiating suprabasal cells. Expression pattern of K8/18 is rather uncommon in mature squamous epithelium.

CKs alterations have been reported in carcinomas from different anatomical sites and these have been associated with specific aspects of tumor behavior.

In the literature, both quantitative and qualitative changes in catenins have been shown to be associated with dedifferentiation, dissemination of tumor cells from primary location, and prognosis in many human tumors. Yet, the exact mechanisms behind changes in the expression of catenin in cancer remains unclear. The actions of catenins in signaling pathways have only been partially clarified, but the most investigated pathway associated with catenins in humans is the so called Wnt signaling pathway. It is demonstrated that oral and lung squamous cell carcinomas express Wnt members and activate the signaling pathway. Identification of Wnt members in normal gingival keratinocytes demonstrates that head and neck carcinoma cells most frequently expressed keratinocyte-type Wnts.

Without Wnt signaling, β-catenin is readily phosphorylated and eventually degraded. The activation of the Wnt signaling pathway may block the turnover of uncomplexed β-catenin, resulting in increased cytoplasmic accumulation.

Chapter 3- Oral squamous cell carcinoma is the most common head and neck cancer and it often has a poor prognosis, owing to local tumor invasion and frequent lymph node metastasis. The development of oral squamous cell carcinoma is usually preceded by a premalignant phase, the most common of which is leukoplakia. Mechanisms of oncogenesis are intimately linked to cell proliferation disruption recognized by intense division and growth, and disturbed maturation. However, for a number of reasons, squamous cell carcinoma is advanced detected, usually when malignant transformation occurred, once it was proved to present specific gene mutation associated. Preceding oral cancer phase, some potentially malignant disorders can appear, marked by alterations in cell kinetics. Herein, the present chapter aims to review the regulation of cell proliferation in development of oral squamous cell carcinoma. Such information plays an important role for understanding the disease, as well as the importance of the detection of preceding oral lesions.

Chapter 4- The squamous cell carcinoma (SCC) arising in epidermal cyst (EC) is a very rare malignant disease but is an enigmatic pathological event and it's hard to find in human pathology a malignancy so surprising and so easy to diagnose. Human papillomavirus associated cyst (HPAC) is a type of epithelial cyst with microscopic features consistent with human papillomavirus (HPV) infection. Only HPV 57 and 60 has been identified in the cystic wall to date. These HPV types are often associated with malignant diseases (high-risk HPV). In this chapter, we describe three cases of SCC arising in epidermal cyst (EC) and the first case of SCC arising in HPAC. Serial sections of all specimens had been prepared in order to verify that the cystic appearance was real and not merely the result of poor orientation of the specimen. In all cases, sections of paraffin-embedded tissue were investigated for the presence of HPV-DNA sequences by polymerase chain reaction (PCR) and *in situ* hybridization. In the first case, an 88-year-old man presented a right zigomatic mass. Histopathology revealed a cyst lined by squamous epithelium in continuity with invasive keratinizing SCC. In the second case, a 96-year-old man consulted your Hospital regard to 1.5x1cm nodule of the right ear's helix. Histopathology showed the typical cystic wall of an EC with transition to invasive keratinizing SCC. In the third case, a 67 year-old man showed ulcerated nodular cystic lesion of the right helix, of 8mm in maximum diameter. Histologically a cystic lesion was lined by squamous epithelium in continuity with invasive SCC. Finally an 86 years-old woman suffered of a perineal cystic nodule of 1.5cm in diameter. Histologically the cystic lesion showed the wall with varying degrees of papillomatosis, hypergranulosis, parakeratosis with dysplastic and koilocytic changes. Areas of *in situ* and invasive SCC were found. Human HPV 16 was detected. Computed tomography with the administration of intravenous contrast material was performed and showed diffuse wall thickening of the anorectum and infiltration of anus muscles' levator. E*ndoscopic biopsies* of *the anal* canal and *rectum* revealed SCC with presence of HPV 16. The patient refused every treatment. Malignant degeneration of EC may be diagnosed only with the support of an accurate histopathological documentation in order to exclude mimics (proliferating epidermal cyst, proliferating trichilemmal cyst). Regarding HPAC, the site, the malignant transformation and the finding of HPV 16 type, may be considered features of an extraordinary rare case

Chapter 5- SCC in the setting of EB is primarily related to RDEB and less often, JEB. It is not related to UV exposure but rather chronic repetitive wounds. The exact mechanism is to be determined but a number of factors have been discovered which may serve as therapeutic targets. Prevention from trauma, to reduce blistering, and early detection by comprehensive examination using digital photography every 3 months, ideally by the same experts, may allow for curative early excision. Some additional therapies, such as tyrosine kinase inhibitors, and retinoids have shown promising results. EB patients can tolerate radiotherapy as an adjunct to surgery. Chemotherapy is a very last resort, due to the risk of sepsis from chronically colonized skin. Research into the cause and better treatments for SCC, the major life threatening complication of RDEB, is one of the highest priorities in EB at present.

Chapter 6- The behavior of nucleolin and AgNOR proteins in ultraviolet (UV) irradiation-induced apoptosis of oral cancer cells was investigated. In addition, the alteration of nucleolin and AgNORs proteins in apoptotic oral cancer cells induced by okadaic acid and anti-cancer drugs in our previous studies was reviewed. Dynamic alterations of nucleolin and AgNORs proteins in UV irradiation-induced apoptotic HSG cells were visualized using Western blot analysis and histocytochemistry methods. It was found that the 110-kDa forms of nucleolin and AgNOR proteins decreased in quantity, while the 80- and 95-kDa forms appeared during apoptosis caused by UV exposure in apoptotic HSG cells. Nucleolin disappeared or diffusely spread out into the nucleus in the apoptotic body of oral cancer cells. Based on this and previous reports, alteration of nucleolin, an AgNOR-associated protein, is associated with the induction of DNA fragmentation in the final active phase of apoptosis in oral cancer cells.

Chapter 7- Tongue is one of the most common sites of oral squamous cell carcinomas (SCC). A good treatment strategy should incorporate an optimal resection with adequate surgical clearance and minimal physical dysfunction. Surgical clearance depends on surgeon's experience as there are no available methods for intraoperative diagnosis. Ultrasonography (US) is increasingly being used in oral and maxillofacial regions for detection of soft tissue-related diseases like salivary gland tumors, regional lymph nodes, etc. US is non-invasive real time imaging technique especially suitable for detecting tumors of small dimensions that are not readable even by CT scan or MRI. At present, US is mainly used as a diagnostic aid. Early stage tongue carcinomas (T1-T2) are especially benefited by US. The use of US before resection of tongue carcinomas for approximate evaluation of tumor thickness is routinely carried out. This time, the authors propose a diagnostic and therapeutic intervention of

US in tongue carcinomas to confirm the surgical clearance and safety margin intraoperatively using a new method.

Chapter 8- *Introduction.* Cuniculatum carcinoma is a well-differentiated form of squamous cell carcinoma that shares histological characteristics with papillary squamous cell carcinoma and verrucous carcinoma. Cuniculatum carcinoma usually occurs on the plantar region, and only few cases involving the oral cavity have been described in the literature.

Methods. A review of the oral cuniculatum carcinoma cases retrieved in the pubmed and google scholar has been performed.

Results. The authors reviewed 19 cases of oral cuniculatum carcinomas. All of the patients were in a great deal of pain. Clinical criteria, osseous lysis and the coexistence of multiple intraosseous well-differentiated, hyperkeratotic papillomatous lesions with few cellular atypies sign the diagnosis. Cervical and distant metastases were rare.

Conclusion. The diagnosis is often delayed because the histological diagnosis may be difficult. Although cuniculatum carcinoma displays aggressive behaviour locally, lymph nodes infiltration and metastasis are rare. The therapy of choice is the surgery alone, after which the prognosis is excellent.

Chapter 9- Imaging of squamous cell carcinoma (SCC) can be a challenging task and usually requires a combination of several imaging modalities that provide different complimentary information about tumor morphology and characterization, as well as indications about tumor prognosis and treatment planning. In this chapter, the role of the various imaging techniques (such as Computed Tomography [CT], Magnetic Resonance Imaging [MRI], and Positron Emission Tomography [PET]) available for the evaluation of head-and-neck SCC will be illustrated, and imaging findings will be discussed along with their correlation with pathologic features. To this purpose, modern multidetector CT technology allows an accurate assessment of tumor extent and morphology owing to its excellent spatial resolution and the possibility to perform 2D and 3D reconstructions of native images with voxel isotropy, while MRI plays a major role for tumor characterization due to its superior contrast resolution and its multiparametric nature. On the other hand, PET can provide metabolic data that are useful for detection of disease recurrence after treatment and lymph node and/or distant dissemination. Particular attention will also be paid to emerging imaging modalities, such as CT perfusion, that can provide functional information about tumor vascularity and represent promising tools for noninvasive evaluation of tumor prognosis before chemo-radiation therapy, as well as of early disease recurrence after treatment.

Chapter 10- Oral cancer is the sixth most common cancer worldwide ahead of Hodgkin's lymphoma, leukemia, brain, stomach, or ovarian cancers, with about 37,000 Americans being diagnosed annually. More than 90% of oral cancers are oral squamous cell carcinomas (OSCC). While the overall 5-year survival rate is about 50%, the survival rate when diagnosed early and treated as localized tumors is as high as 90%. Currently the gold standard for diagnosis of OSCC is early visual detection of a suspicious oral lesion followed by scalpel biopsy with adjunct histology. However, there are multiple limitations associated with biopsies: being invasive clinicians are hesitant to perform them, and patients may not agree to them due to the pain and discomfort of the procedure; the following histology requires expert analysis and is therefore expensive; and issues such as under-sampling add uncertainty to diagnosis. An ideal alternative to scalpel biopsy would be non-invasively collected samples containing biomarkers which can distinguish between oral pre-malignant lesions (OPMLs) and OSCC, and potentially predict the transition from pre-malignancy to malignancy. Methods for sampling and discovering biomarkers of OSCC in a non-invasive fashion have been emerging, including those focusing on whole saliva and cells and other specimens collected directly from oral lesions. These samples are ideally suited for system-wide analysis using genomic and proteomic technologies for biomarker discovery. Here, the authors describe the current state of the clinical diagnosis of oral cancer, with an emphasis on emerging genomic and proteomic strategies seeking to identify non-invasively collected biomarkers that could improve the early diagnosis of OPML transition to OSCC.

Chapter 11- Background: The mutated p53 and p21 is believed to play a major role in tumorigenesis including oral cancer. The purpose of this study was to determine whether there is an evidence of field cancerization based on the profile of p53 and p21 expression in normal oral mucosa adjacent to restricted squamous cell carcinomas.

Materials and Methods: Immunehistochemistry for p53 and p21 was performed in fresh frozen samples of morphologically normal oral mucosa taken from 34 cancer patients (NC) and 21 non-cancer patients (NN). Stained sections were assessed and the results were analysed using Minitab 13.1 statistical package.

Results: P53 and p21 expressions were found to be positive in 20 (58.8%) and 22 (64.7%) cases of the NC group respectively, and in 8 (38%) and 8 (38%) cases of the NN group respectively. When the results of both groups

were compared the difference was found to be statistically significant
(P<0.05). P53 expression was found to be higher in the NC biopsies taken
from patients with poorly differentiated compared to well differentiated SCCs
(P=0.034) and with or without second tumour (P=0.052).

Conclusion: The authors conclude that the differences in the expression of
p53 and p21 in NC compared NN groups, as well as the higher expression of
p53 in the NC with poorly differentiated SCC and the possibility of getting a
second tumour may be considered as a marker of field cancerization.

Chapter 12- The treatment alternatives for squamous cell carcinoma of the
glottic and supraglottic larynx are discussed. The optimal treatment depends
on the location and extent of the primary tumor, presence and extent of
clinically postive nodes, and the medical condition of the patient. Treatment
selection is addressed and the outcomes after radiotherapy and/or surgery are
presented

In: Squamous Cell Carcinoma   ISBN: 978-1-61209-929-3
Editor: Daniel V. Mortensen   © 2012 Nova Science Publishers, Inc.

Chapter 1

SQUAMOUS CELL CARCINOMA ONTOGENY: PART I

S. Díaz Prado[1,2], V. Medina Villaamil[2],
G. Aparicio Gallego[2], R. García Campelo[3]
and L.M. Anton Aparicio[1,3]

[1]Medicine Department. Universitario of A Coruña, A Coruña, Spain
[2]INIBIC-Hospital Universitario A Coruña, A Coruña, Spain
[3]Medical Oncology Service. Hospital Universitario A Coruña,
A Coruña, Spain

ABSTRACT

Populations of cancer stem cells (CSCs) have been found and characterized in multiple malignancies as many cancers; however, this has not fully happened yet in human squamous cell carcinomas (SCC) of the lung, cervix and head & neck.

The field of stem cell biology is growing and will result in the steady identification of multi-potent, self-renewing, and proliferative progenitor's cell populations. These cells give rise to both transiently amplifying (TA) and terminally differentiated (TD) cells, which are important for tissue maintenance.

In leukemia, for example, it has been shown that partially committed cells, which are normally responsible for tissue maintenance after trauma may undergo transformation via mutations resulting in the selective expression of genes that accentuate and perpetuate these cells' self-renewal capabilities.

Bearing this in mind, it is valid to view stem cells as pro-tumorigenic. It has been proposed that the accumulation of oncogenic events may *lock* activated stem cells in a permanent aberrant state, which converts normal homeostatic stem cells into *cancer stem cells*. Because many developmental signaling pathways drive these cells into neoplasia, we are required to understand. in some detail. their intricacies.

The observation that the earlier stage of human organ development to which a human tumor resembled was linked with worse survival rates suggested that abnormally-activated embryological cell signaling pathways are important in carcinogenesis. In order for an organism to develop, its cells need to be able to proliferate and to follow specific fates of cellular differentiation in a tightly controlled temporospatial manner, to ultimately ensemble and organize into functioning tissue and organs. Cell fate specification and complex gene regulatory networks (GRN) control development.

Cellular phenotypes are the result of patterns of gene expression. Intrinsic transcription factors released by cells in a timely manner provide the coordinates that delineate their individual fate. Extrinsic factors influence cells as groups through the process of differentiation. The integration of intrinsic and extrinsic cues is the decisive denominator, providing the coordinates of cell fate and differentiation. By understanding the interplay between these factors, we will hopefully dissect the processes leading to cell fate assignment.

As we continue to understand, in detail, the repercussions of deregulation in key embryonic signaling pathways, we begin to dissect their intricate relationships with the stem cells and malignancy. We can explain how aberrations inflicted in many of the components of this complex homeostatic engine can lead to the formation of cancer stem cells with accumulated permanent mutations that allow them to re-populate their tumors rendering these lesions.

Research data from the last two decades suggests that there are four main signaling transduction pathways in the cell: Wnt, Hedgehog, Notch, and Bone morphogenic proteins. They are thought to act in parallel, to ultimately enhance specific genes that results in cell type-specific combinations of transcription factors responsible for cellular behavior, representing the basic machinery for determination of embryonic cell fate determination.

In this chapter, we explore the roles of the main developmental signaling pathways in organogenesis and maintenance, together with the issue of homeostatic stem cells within specific *niches* in the lung and maxillofacial tract. The aim, of course, is to ultimately integrate the knowledge of these mechanisms into tangible tools that can be eventually translated into novel therapies against the human cancers.

1. ORIGIN OF CANCER

In 1889, Sir S. Paget introduced the *soil and seed* hypothesis of metastasis to medicine, by crediting the idea to Fuchs (Fuchs, 1882). In Paget's study, he concludes that the distribution of metastases cannot be due to chance alone and that different tissues provide optimal conditions for the growth of specific cancers (Paget, 1889).

In the *soil and seed* metaphor, the *soil* refers to the secondary site of tumor growth and development, and perhaps the chemical signals produced in the micro-environment at the potential sites of metastasis (Langley & Fidler, 2007; Strieter, 2001). The *seed* is the ostensible stem cell or tumor-initiating cell from the primary tumor (Chung et al., 2005) These tumor-initiating cells are the tumorigenic farce behind tumor initiation, growth, metastasis, drug resistance, and relapse (reviewed in Pardal et al., 2003).

In a variation of this idea, called the *homing* hypothesis, a secondary signal secreted by cells at the future metastatic sites *calls* the tumor cells and permits them to proliferate there (Hewitt et al., 2000; Stetler-Stevenson, 2001). In this hypothesis, the *seed* produces cell surface receptors able to recognize the site demarcated by the *soil*. Although the mechanisms of tissue specificity remain obscure, researchers have focused on small messenger molecules as attractants and larger cell surface receptors guiding the tumor-initiating cells or *seeds*. Muller (Müller et al., 2001) and Murphy (Murphy, 2001) have each focused on chemokines and their receptors as viable candidates for *soil and seed* signaling. Murphy specifically proposes a "spatial and temporal code" made up of specific combinations of such molecules, and other being responsible for neovascularization, metastasis, and immunosurveillance avoidance.

1.1. Oncogenes

Proto-oncogene is a normal gene that can become an oncogene due to mutations or increased *expression*. The resultant protein may be termed an oncoprotein. Proto-oncogenes code for *proteins* that help to regulate *cell growth* and *differentiation*. Proto-oncogenes are often involved in *signal transduction* and the execution of *mitogenic* signals, usually through their *protein* products. Upon activation, a proto-oncogene (or its product) becomes a tumor-inducing agent, an oncogene.

There are two mechanisms by which proto-oncogenes can be converted to cellular oncogenes:

Quantitative: Tumor formation is induced by an increase in the absolute number of proto-oncogene products or by its production in inappropriate cell types.

Qualitative: Conversion from proto-oncogene to transforming gene (c-onc) with changes in the nucleotide sequence which are responsible for the acquisition of the new properties.

A concept of the oncogene appeared in the early 1970s (Zilber et al., 1975). Several studies of tumorigenic retroviruses have revealed a whole family of oncogenes with different activities and action mechanisms from MGCV (mammary gland cancer virus of low oncogenicity) of mice to RSV (Rous sarcoma virus). Oncogenes demonstrated an elementary carcinogenesis determined by a *single* mutant gene.

A tumorigenic DNA virus cannot capture a proto-oncogene and is free of classic oncogenes. Genes responsible for tumors induced by DNA viruses have another mechanism of action and another origin. Their tumorigenic activity is not determined by the cellular proto-oncogene incorporated into the virus structure.

Oncogenes are structural components of oncogenic oncornaviruses and can be identified and characterized by comparing them with the structure of the initial (non-oncogenic) viruses. In such a manner the main groups of viral oncogenes were established (*SRC, RAS, ABL, MYC, SIS*) and shown to occur on different stages of signaling pathways, from growth signal-specific receptors, such as PDGF (*SIS* oncogene) to oncogenes acting inside the cell (*RAS, SRC*) or within the nucleus (*MYC*) where they activate a specific gene group as transcription factors (Tatosyan et al., 2004). The signal specificity is determined by changes in the conformation of all preceding links activated by their ligands.

The viral antigen located in the signal transduction chain and not needing an initial ligand (growth factor or hormone) generates mitogenic signals into the nucleus and thus determines the autonomous proliferation of the cell. Signals from oncogenes are dominant. They need no homozygosity because the viral oncogene is beyond regulation as not being a part of the normal genome. Certainly, it should be remembered that the transmission of a mitogenic signal from the oncogene into the nucleus includes many intermediate stages and crosses other signaling pathways.

Hemoblastoses, or tumors of the hemopoietic system, are caused by one oncogene, a proto-oncogene (i.e. their own gene), activated by translocation under the promoter of a physiologically-active gene, or by mutation of one proto-oncogene. In most cases (if not always), they are dominant, and all known manifestations of such oncogenes are dominant or co-dominant, e.g. BCR (B-cellular, i.e. immunoglobulin receptor)–ABL or IgG-MYC (Fleishman, 2007). The oncogenic effect of an activated proto-oncogene is obviously dominant.

This is responsible for a fundamental difference of human carcinomas and hemoblastoses. Human carcinomas are always, or in the great majority of cases, induced by usually recessive tumor suppressor genes and combined oncogenic actions of several proto-oncogenes, whereas in the case of hemoblastoses, a single activated dominant proto-oncogene is acting, which needs involvement of additional genes only to enhance the effect, as a rule, during tumor progression.

The path of hemoblastoses to malignancy is much shorter and easier than the path of carcinomas; therefore, it is not surprising that carcinomas usually require an interaction of a number of independent oncogenes (Hanahan y Weinberg, 2000). Activation of proto-oncogenes due to translocation frequently occurs in hemoblastoses, and is classically exemplified by translocation of the gene, *ABL,* under the gene BCR promoter (Ph-chromosome) in chronic myelocytic leukemia. However, in hemoblastoses, it is not always clear how, when, and in what cell population the crisis comes.

Hemoblastoses are more elementary systems than carcinomas, which, in particular, are determined by direct intercellular interactions (not mediated through cytokines), direct interactions with extracellular matrix, and by acquisition of invasion and metastasis via selection for autonomicity, which is an essence of progression.

Another fundamental distinction should also be mentioned: hemoblastoses retain the normal phenotype of the cell precursor as a mechanism involved in proto-oncogene activation (Abelev, 2007). These features make hematopoietic tumors extraordinarily similar to the precursor cells.

The differentiation characteristics of hemoblastoses are seriously different from those of carcinomas. When carcinomas can more or less lose features of their tissue differentiation, hemoblastoses retain their differentiation until the transformation stage. The transformation seems to correspond to "motionless" of the differentiation, and this allows us to finely classify hemoblastoses and determine their origin. This occurs because the majority of hemoblastoses are a result of chromosomal translocations, when the role of an "activating" gene is played by the gene actively expressed in the tissue under consideration (e.g. *BCR*), and the differentiation block is determined by an unrelated "activated" gene located on a fragment of the translocated chromosome (e.g. *ABL*). This unrelated gene acts as an "oncogene", which inhibits the differentiation and determines a pathologic autonomous proliferation. It is single and dominant, i.e. acts as an oncogene. Additional mutations can enhance or accelerate its action but are not components of its oncogenic effect.

1.2. Two-Hit Hypothesis

It has been proposed that the two-hit hypothesis explains the early onset at multiple sites in the body of an inherited form of cancer called hereditary retinoblastoma. Inheriting one germ line copy of a damaged gene present in every cell in the body was not sufficient to enable this cancer to develop. A second hit (or loss) to the good copy in the gene pair could occur somatically though, producing cancer. This hypothesis predicted that the chances for a germ line mutation carrier to get a second somatic mutation at any of the multiple sites in his/her body cells was much greater than the chances for a non-carrier to get two hits in the same cell.

Knudson suggested that multiple "hits" to DNA were necessary to cause cancer. In the children with inherited retinoblastoma, the first insult was inherited in the DNA, and any second insult would rapidly lead to cancer. In non-inherited retinoblastoma, two "hits" had to take place before a tumor could develop, explaining the age difference.

It was later found that *carcinogenesis* (the development of malignancy) depended both on the activation of *proto-oncogenes* (genes that stimulate cell proliferation) and deactivation of *tumor suppressor genes* (genes that keep proliferation in check). A first "hit" in an oncogene would not necessarily lead to cancer, as normally functioning tumor suppressor genes (TSGs) would still counterbalance this impetus; only damage to TSGs would lead to unchecked proliferation. Conversely, a damaged TSG (such as the Rb1 gene in retinoblastoma) would not lead to cancer unless there is a growth impetus from an activated oncogene.

Field cancerization may be an extended form of the Knudson hypothesis. This is the phenomenon of various primary tumors developing in one particular area of the body, suggesting that an earlier "hit" predisposed the whole area for malignancy.

Unlike oncogenes, tumor suppressor genes generally follow the 'two-hit hypothesis', which implies that both alleles that code for a particular gene must be affected before an effect is manifested. This is due to the fact that if only one allele for the gene is damaged, the second can still produce the correct protein. In other words, mutant tumor suppressors' alleles are usually recessive, whereas mutant oncogene alleles are typically dominant. Oncogene mutations, in contrast, generally involve a single allele because they gain function mutations. There are notable exceptions to the 'two-hit' rule for tumor suppressors, such as certain mutations in the p53 gene product. p53 mutations can function as a 'dominant negative', meaning that a mutated p53 protein can prevent the function of normal protein from the un-mutated allele. Other tumor-suppressor genes that are exceptions to the 'two-hit' rule are those that exhibit haploinsufficiency for example PTCH in medulloblastoma. An example of this is the p27Kip1 cell-cycle inhibitor, in which mutation of a single allele causes increased carcinogen susceptibility.

1.3. Initiation and Promotion

The notion of cancer initiation and promotion came from the models of chemical carcinogenes. According to these models, the initiation event causes genetic damage in a pre-malignant cell, and the promotional factors stimulate the damaged cell to become cancerous and proliferate (Yaamagiwa & Ichiikawa, 1918; Kennaway, 1955; Rous & Kidd, 1942; Berenblum & Shubick, 1947). Chemical benzopyrene in skin cells, through binding to DNA, caused permanent genetic alterations (intiation) but cancer would not form unless another stimulus was applied to affected skin (promotion) (Friedwald & Rous, 1944).

Three major theories of cancer (somatic mutation, virus causation, and faulty differentiation) are proposed to involve alterations in DNA structure. Each results in terms of failures in the normal intercellular communication that involves feedback between differentiated cells acting on less differentiated cells still capable of proliferation. The historical background of the latter idea is traced to Osgood, Weiss and Kavanau, and to Iversen. The historical background of concepts of initiation and promotion are traced to Berenblum and Mottram and the Boutwell concept of promotion as gene activation is cited. It is proposed that gene activation by promoters is a valid concept and that it results from the blocking of the normal intercellular communication postulated by Osgood and others. The problem of explaining the low probability of cancer following initiators or promoters acting alone is cited as a problem in basic science. A hypothesis to solve the problem is proposed: cancer results from two of more relevant mutations: promoters enhance proliferation of cells with one relevant mutation, thereby increasing the probability of obtaining a cell with two relevant mutations.

The initial experimental studies of carcinogenesis were conducted in animals. Chemicals able to react with DNA and non-reactive compounds were both tested for their ability to cause cancer. The model used was mouse skin carcinogenesis. In this system, researchers painted test chemicals on the skin and observed the growth of tumors. Researchers found that the application of a DNA-reactive substance only resulted in tumor formation when the animals were further treated with another non-reactive substance. A compound that reacts with DNA and somehow changes the genetic makeup of the cell is called a mutagen. The mutagens that predispose cells to develop tumors are called initiators and the non-reactive compounds that stimulate tumor development are called promoters. Approximately 70% of known mutagens are also carcinogens--cancer-causing compounds. A compound that acts as both an initiator and a promoter is referred to as a 'complete carcinogen' because tumor development can occur without the application of another compound. Initiation is the first step in the two-stage model of cancer development. Initiators, if not already reactive with DNA, are altered (frequently they are made electrophilic) via drug-metabolizing enzymes in the body and are then able to cause changes in DNA (mutations). Since many initiators must be metabolized before becoming active, initiators are often specific to particular tissue types or species. The effects of initiators are irreversible; once a particular cell has been affected by an initiator, it is susceptible to promotion until its death. Since initiation is the result of permanent genetic change, any daughter cells produced from the division of the mutated cell will also carry the mutation. In studies of mouse skin carcinogenesis, a linear relationship has been observed between the dose of initiator and the quantity of tumors that can be produced, thus any exposure to the initiator increases risk and this risk increases indefinitely with higher levels of exposure.

Once a cell has been mutated by an initiator, it is susceptible to the effects of promoters. These compounds promote the proliferation of the cell, giving rise to a large number of daughter cells containing the mutation created by the initiator. Promoters have no effect when the organism in question has not been previously treated with an initiator.

Unlike initiators, promoters do not covalently bind to DNA or macromolecules within the cell. Many bind to receptors on the cell surface in order to affect intracellular pathways that lead to increased cell proliferation. There are two general categories of promoters: specific promoters that interact with receptors on or in target cells of defined tissues and non-specific promoters that alter gene expression without the presence of a known receptor. Promoters are often specific for a particular tissue or species due to their interaction with receptors that are present in different amounts in different tissue types.

While the risk of tumor growth with promoter application is dose-dependent, there is both a threshold and a maximum effect of promoters. Very low doses of promoters will not lead to tumor development and extremely high doses will not produce more risk than moderate levels of exposure.

1.4. Multi-step Carcinogenesis

The multi-step model of carcinogenesis holds that the development of cancer is a multi-step process in which exposure to carcinogens results in repeated damage and repair. Eventually, the accumulated exposure triggers a transformation from normal to pre-malignant cells (i.e., from normal cells to metaplasia and dysplasia) and eventually to carcinoma. Multi-step carcinogenesis on the molecular level is best described in colon cancer (Lengauer et al., 1998).

A genetic model for multi-step carcinogenesis caused for field cancerization has been described (Braakhuis et al., 2003). A stem cell acquires one or more genetic mutations and forms a cluster of cells with genetically altered progeny cells. Accumulated genetic alterations then leads to dysregulation of stem cell growth causing clonal expansion (Vogelstein & Kinsler, 1993). This creates a *field lesion* which displaces normal epithelium. Further proliferation at the accelerated growth rate enables additional genetic hits to occur and can lead to numerous subclones within the field lesion. These subclones can then take divergent pathways depending on the respective accumulated genetic abnormalities (Tabor et al., 2001). Eventually, a subclone will evolve into a malignancy and accumulate other independent events which can lead to metastatic disease (Califano et al., 1999).

2. CANCER STEM CELL THEORY

2.1. Field Cancerization

The concept of field cancerization was first introduced (Slaugther et al., 1953) after noting the presence of multiple *independent* tumors and *abnormal epithelium* in the mucosa adjacent to head and neck squamous cell carcinomas (HNSCC). That report postulated that *multi-centric origin through a process of field cancerization would seem to be an important factor in the persistence or recurrence of epidermoid carcinoma following therapy*. In its classical interpretation, the concept of field cancerization refers to large areas of the aerodigestive tract mucosa affected by long term exposure to carcinogens, resulting in genetically altered fields in which multi-focal carcinomas can develop because of independent genetic events.

The carcinogenic link between smoking and lung cancer development can be explained in terms of two concepts: field carcinogenesis and the model of multi-step carcinogenesis. (Auerbach et al., 1957; Slaugther et al., 1953). Genetic changes, pre-malignant and malignant lesions in one region of the field translate into an increased risk of cancer development in the entire field. Areas of carcinoma *in situ* and metaplasia have been found to occur in the bronchial epithelium after prolonged exposure to inhaled carcinogenic agents, specifically cigarette smoke. There is increasing molecular evidence that these areas of histologic change are causally related to the development of lung cancer (Auerbach et al., 1979 & 1961).

The term of field cancerization, a condition in which the mucosa is primed to the development of multiple and independent transformation events as consequences of carcinogenes, describe a situation in which: a) oral cancer develops in multi-focal areas of pre-cancerous change; b) histologically abnormal tissue surrounds the tumor; c) oral cancer often consists of multiple independent lesions that sometimes coalesce; and d) the persistence of abnormal tissue after surgery may explain second primary tumors and local recurrences (Slaugther et al., 1953, Braakhuis et al., 2005).

2.2. Field Cancerization, Multi-focal Disease, and Second Malignancies

The development of locally recurrent cancer and second primary tumors in patients can be explained by the concept of field cancerization (Slaugther et al., 1953). Although there is substantial molecular and genetic evidence supporting the concept of field cancerization, debate remains over the clonal relation of pre-neoplastic and neoplastic lesions developing in these fields and their mode of spread (Forastiere et al., 2001). Establishing the clonal relation of multiple tumors in the same patient is not always easy or straightforward. Unrelated tumors may lose the same allele by chance alone, and related tumors may show differing allelotypes allowing the accumulation of new alterations during tumor progression.

In fact, recent studies have identified small clusters, *patches*, of genetically aberrant cells in the squamous epithelium. Such a *patch* has been interpreted as a clonal unit of altered cells, and it has been proposed that a p53 mutated patch within the epithelium could be considered as the very first manifestation of carcinogenesis (Braakhuis et al., 2005; Mackenzie, 2004; Moolgavkar & Luebeck, 2003; Perez-Losada & Balmain, 2003; Rajagopalan et al., 2003).

2.3. Field Cancerization and Stem Cells

The biology of stem cells and their properties have already been recognized as integral to tumor pathogenesis in several types of cancer. A role for stem cells has been demonstrated for the hematopoietic system diseases, breast and brain cancers (Jordan, 2004). Going forward, it seems that the possible involvement of stem cells in other malignancies will also be clarified, including head and neck tumors and lung cancer. This model has been proposed for head and neck cancer that should originate from aberrant stem cells within the epithelium/mucosa (Owens & Watt, 2003).

For cancer development, it has been proposed that a stem cell acquires one (or more) genetic alterations, and forms a *patch* in the mucosal epithelium with genetically altered daughter cells. As a result of this process, cancer stem cell scapes the normal control mechanisms and gains growth advantage: the *patch* starts to expand and a tumor develops. In this way, areas of formal epithelium can be replaced by cell populations that become increasingly more genetically altered cells which is considered as a serious risk and at a certain malignant clone (Forastiere &Koch, 2001).

It is recognized that cancers contain subpopulations of cancer cells that often resemble the developmental hierarchy of normal tissues from which the cancer develops. Until recently, the importance of the cancer cell subpopulations to tumor development and growth has been poorly understood. The identification of small subpopulations of highly tumorigenic cancer cells in a variety of solid human tumors has stimulated great interest in the cancer stem-cell (CSC) theory of tumorigenesis.

According to the CSC theory, only a specific subpopulation of cancer cells have the ability to sustain cancer growth, and all of the other cancer cells have a limited growth potential or no growth potential at all.

2.4. The Concept of Field Cancerization *versus* Cancer Stem Cells

The identification of cancer stem cells in head and neck tumors represents a fundamental goal in the agenda of stem cell biologists as well as the detection of the key factors involved in self-renewal and differentiation pathways.

Recently, human head and neck squamous cell cancers contain a tumorigenic, so-called cancer stem cell, subpopulation of cells that can self-renew and produce differentiated cells that form the bulk of the tumor. These tumorigenic HHSCC cells have a distinct phenotype and can be identified by a surface marker (Prince et al., 2007). These cells are comprised of a small population of the HNSCC cells, usually less than 10%; they can be separated from the other cancer cells with the surface marker CD44; could self-renew; and could reproduce the original tumor heterogeneity (Mackenzie, 2004; Prince & Ailles, 2008). Analysis by flow cytometry revealed that HNSCC tumor cells were heterogeneous for CD44 expression. The cancer cells with a high expression of the cell surface marker CD44 had significant tumorigenic potential. The CD44$^+$ subpopulation of cells produced more tumors that CD44$^-$ subpopulations cells. Although the CD44$^+$ head and neck squamous cell carcinoma cells are capable of producing new tumors, the relatively high number that must be implanted to induce tumor growth led us to hypothesize that this subpopulation of cells did not represent a *pure* population of head and neck squamous cell carcinoma CSCs. These findings provide further evidence that HNSCC is organized into a developmental hierarchy, as it is predicted by the CSC theory of carcinogenesis.

The identification of a population of highly tumorigenic cells in HNSCC with the exclusive ability to produce new tumors and re-create the original tumor heterogeneity is a significant advancement in the study of HNSCC. When viewed in combination with other work reporting the identification of CSCs in other tumor types, it provides further evidence supporting the validity of the CSC theory of carcinogenesis. There are sufficient evidences supporting both the *old cancer model*, considering the cancer as a proliferative disease and the *new cancer model*, considering the cancer as a stem cell disorder or a disease of unregulated self-renewal and not as a simple mechanism whereby cell proliferation is disrupted.

3. STEM CELLS

3.1. Stem Cells Concept

A normal stem cell (SC) is defined by its ability to continually re-populate the cells that comprise the organ system in which they exist. Three properties that enable a stem cell to do this are its differentiation capability (pluripotency), the ability to self-renewal (Figure 1), and a high proliferative capacity (reviewed in Tang et al., 2007). The ability of a normal SC to support and propagate an organ or tissue must be tightly regulated.

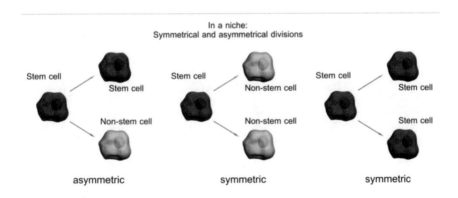

Figure 1. Symmetrical and asymmetrical divisions of a stem cell in a niche.

Most stem cells in the body remain in a dormant state. These cells are surrounded by other, differentiated cells within the tissue microenvironment often described as a *niche*. The cells of the niche regulate the stem cells via cell-cell contacts, interactions with the extracellular matrix, and secretion of inhibitory factors. The disruption of the niche microenvironment, through infection, inflammation, tissue damage, or chemical assault, can activate the division of the stem cells.

A stem cell wil give rise to a number of different cell types that can be broken down into three groups: fully differentiated cells, transit-amplifying cells, and stem cells (reviewed in Stingl & Caldas, 2007). The fully differentiated cells are mitotically inactive cells. They are at the end-stages of cellular differentiation and will never re-enter the active cell cycle phase. The transit-amplifying (TA) cells are fast growing cells that are not fully differentiated. TA cells are able to proliferate for several generations but they eventually terminally differentiate and need to be replenished by the SC. Pluripotency is the ability of a SC to differentiate into the heterogeneous population of cells that are comprised of a tissue or, in the case of cancer stem cell (CSCs), a tumor (reviewed in Lobo et al., 2007).

3.2. Finding Stem Cells

3.2.1. The Airways Stem Cells

Stem cell research in the lung has progressed rather slowly due to anatomical and functional complexities associated with numerous distinct cell types (Anton Aparicio & Díaz Prado, 2007). This organ must be divided into various anatomical regions when considering multi-potent progenitor or stem cells.

Table I. Stem or progenitor cells characteristics in airway

Tissue	Epitheliam stem cell niche	Daughter cells
Lung proximal	Tracheal basal cell	Mucous, ciliated neuroendocrine
	Tracheal mucous-gland duct cell	Mucous, ciliated neuroendocrine
	Tracheal secretory cell	Mucous, ciliated, neuroendocrine
Distal	Bronchiolar Clara cell	Mucous, ciliated neuroendocrine
	Alveolar type II pneumocyte	Type I & II pneumocyte (Clara cells)
	Neuroendocrine	PNEC & Clara cells

Evidence clearly suggests that multi-potent progenitors of the conducting airway epithelium and gas-exchange alveolar regions are derived from different populations of stem ells that are anatomically separated in the lung. Stem cell niches in the conducting airways must also be uniquely divided between the proximal and distal regions (Aparicio Gallego et al., 2007) (Table I).

Bronchial airways harbor at least two distinct progenitor cell populations. Both basal and non-ciliated secretory cell types of bronchial airways have been shown to exibit proliferative capacity. The disparity between bronchial and bronchiolar airways is consistent with a mechanism in which the actvity of distint progenitor cell pools accounts for regional differences in both lineage specifications during lung development and in the cellular composition of tracheobronchial and bronchiolar airways.

Epithelia cell composition and zone boundaries depend on both the species and the individual animal history. In normal mice, a renewing cell system encompasing a gland-containing, pseudostratified epithelium with Clara cells and few globet cells is present in the upper trachea, whereas in humans, this zone penetrates many bronchial generations. Distally, the airway epithelium becomes glandless and cuboidal. It is dominated by a Clara cell-based lineage system before its transformation into a type II cell-based system in the alveoli.

Stem cell niches in the airways have been characterized through experiments with rodent models. The proximal mouse trachea resides in the submucous gland duct, whereas those from the bronchioles come from a subset of cells expressing Clara-cell-specific protein located near neuroendocrine bodies and broncho-alveolar-duct junction. This variation in the structure of airway epithelium has raised many interrogants regarding the probable location/origin for a stem cells niche. In the airway, however, specific niches of stem cell expansion have been identified and marked by distinct zonal boundaries. In the proximal glandular containing the trachea, label-retaining cells (LRC) expanding zones were confined to the ducts of sub-mucosal glands, while in more distal trachea and bronchi, which do not contain glands, these LRC expanding stem cells were located in systematically arrayed foci along the surface airway epithelium. These foci in the distal tranchea also appeared to be localized at cartilage-intercartilage junctions. Distal tracheal foci of LCRs tended to correspond with the position of the cartilage-intercartilage junction where blood vessels and nerves typically penetrate toward the epithelial surface, where gland rudiments were occasionallty observed, and were frequently present in the surface epithelium.

These studies clearly demonstrated that regeneration surface airway epithelium could emerge from gland ducts and supports the notion that this region may be a stem cell niche. In the distal non-glandular trachea and distal bronchiolar airways, similar niches for LCR were seen following transit amplifying cells (TA) ablation.

The existence of multiple progenitor cell types within the bronchial epithelium and hierarchy with which they participate in epithelial maintenance is of fundamental importance to epithelial remodeling. The primitive pluripotent epithelial cells that formate the lung have the potential to form both the bronchial and the alveolar-cell lineages (Figure 2). It is not known whether there are any stem cells in the developed lung that could give rise to both airway and alveolar epithelial cells. Both the airway and the alveolar compartment have a transiently dividing compartment of differentiated epithelial cells.

PULMONARY EPITHELIAL CELL LINEAGES

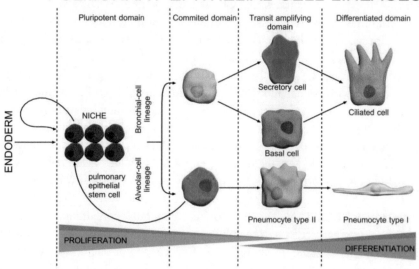

Figure 2. A conceptual diagram of epithelial lineages in the lung. Stem cells renew themselves indefinitely as well as producing transit-amplifying cells.

3.2.2. The Oral Stem Cells

Post-natal stem cells have been isolated from various tissues, including dental epithelium (Harada et al., 1999) , dental pulp (Gronthos et al., 2002 & 2000), and their differentiation is regulated by various potent regulators of bone formation, including members of the TGFβ superfamily and cytokines (Kettunen et al., 1998).

Experiments suggests that the stem cells for differentiated dental epithelium reside in the cervical loop, consisting of a central core of stellate reticulum cells surrounded by a layer of basal epithelial cells, and they give rise to transit-amplifying progeny differentiating into enamel forming ameloblasts (Harada et al., 1999, Tummers & Thesleff, 2003).

In the labial cervical loop, the epithelial stem cells proliferate and migrate along the labial surface, diffentiating into enamel-forming ameloblasts (Klein et al., 2008). In contrast, the ligual cervical loop contains fewer proliferating stem cells (Wang et al., 2007).

Many adult tissues contain tissue-specific stem cells and there are reports that these stem cells were sparsely present along the basal compartment, and not in a certain limited area in the basal layer; each column generated by a single stem cell was called an *epidermal proliferative unit (EPU)* (Ghazizadeh & Taichman, 2005).

Similar to that in the epidermis, there might be proliferative units for renewal of the oral mucosal epithelium (Li et al., 1998; Hakeyama et al., 2007).

Three types of anatomically distinct epithelial are associated with the dentogingival junction, namely the junctional, sulcular, and oral gingival epithelia (Freeman, 1998).The keratinizing oral gingival epithelium lines the external surface, while the non-keratinizing sulcular epithelium lines the inner sulcus. The junctional epithelium, which collars the tooth, has cellular characteristics different from those of the other two epithelia, such as the types of keratin (Freeman, 1998) and adhesion molecules (Hatakeyama et al., 2006).

The basal layers of the oral epithelium contain cells with self-renewing capacity. This population of stem cells contributes to the physiological renewal of the epithelium lining the oral cavity and tongue, and contributes to its rapid regeneration upon damage (Costea et al., 2006). As these stem cells are the only keratinocytes that would reside long enough to accumulate the number of mutations observed in oral cancers, it is highly likely that HNSCC may arise from the malignant transformation of cells within the stem cells niche, or form more differentiated cells that have recovery self-renewing capacity (Costea et al., 2006).

3.3. Cancer Stem Cells

A malignant tumor is composed of a heterogeneous population of cells with varying degrees of tumorigenic potential, and only a subset of cancer cells can initiate and propagate a tumor.

Cancer can be thought of as a disease resulting from the abnormal growth of stem cell, resulting from chronic activation of stem cells (caused by disruptuion of the niche) and leading to the long-term proliferation of the stem cells.

A cancer stem cell (CSC) requires these same properties to sustain and spread a tumor. However, a CSC would not be subjected to the same type of genetic regulation as a normal SC (reviewed in Clarke, 2005). It is also noteworthy that the term *cancer stem cell* does not necessarily imply that its origins are from a SC, as there is the possibility that CSCs emerge from early, less-differentiated cells, committed populations.

These observations led investigators to hypothesize that the clonogenic cells arose from CSCs that maintain the rest of the population. However, the stochastic model of tumorigenesis was equally plausible.

The stochastic model states that all cancer cells can proliferate extensively, from colonies *in vitro*, and initiate new tumors, but only a small fraction has the probability of finding a permissive environment, or niche, for tumor growth (Huntly & Gilliland, 2005; Perryman & Sylvester, 2006). In contrast, the cancer stem cell model posits that most cancer cells are unable to proliferate extensively, cannot form colonies *in vitro*, and are unable to initiate new tumors (reviewed in Wicha et al., 2006).

Insights into the function and characteristic of CSCs will be to offer a novel approach to understanding the progression of metastasis: given that a single cancer cell can drive the formation of a metastatic tumor (Fidler & Talmadge, 1986), CSCs are likely responsible for distant tumorigenesis as they are in primary tumor formation. Thus, research focused on the role of CSCs in primary lesions has lead to the discovery that CSCs can drive tumor formation in leukemia as well as various solid tumors. While little work has been done to elucidate the role of CSCs in metastasis, properties of CSCs such as self-renewal and differentiation make them logical candidates for metastatic colonizers. To facilitate the discussion of CSCs with different metastatic ability, a distinction should be made referring to two potential subtypes of CSCs: primary tumor cancer stem cells (pCSCs) and metastatic cancer stem cells (mCSCs). The first, pCSCs, constitute the original population of tumorigenic cells which initiate the formation of the hematopoietic and solid tumors, and are the center of most CSCs. The second group, mCSCs, represent a distinct population of cells with the intrinsic properties to disseminate from the primary site and generate the distant metastases.

Though other cell subpopulations may break free of the primary tumor and invade the blood stream, mCSCs, like their pCSCs counterparts, are those solely responsible for the initiation of tumors. mCSCs are related to pCSCs in essential properties of self-renewal and differentiation needed for the propagation of the bulk of the tumor, but differ in key ways. Unlike pCSCs, mCSCs disseminate from the tumor, colonize foreign tissue, and likely have additional alterations (whether mutational, epigenetic, or adaptative) which allow survival and propagation in secondary sites.

Key characteristics define the CSC subpopulations: 1) only a small portion of the cancer cells within a tumor have tumorigenic potential when transplanted into immunodeficient mice; 2) the CSC subpopulation can be separated from the other cancer cells by distinctive cell surface markers; 3) tumors resulting from the CSCs contain the mixed tumorigenic and non-tumorigenic cells of the original tumor; and 4) the CSC subpopulation can be serially transplanted through multiple generations, indicating that it is a self-renewing population (Brennan et al., 1995; Costea et al., 2006; Chan et al., 1999).

3.3.1. Stem Cells and Lung Cancer

Classically, the stem/progenitor cells of the pulmonary epithelium are considered to be the basal in the proximal airways, Clara cells in the bronchioles and type II pneumocytes in the alveoli. In the trachea and bronchi, the basal cells are widely believed to be stem cells (Bishop, 2003; Emura, 2002 & 1997; Gazdar et al., 1990, Giangreco et al., 2002). The basal cells, and the parabasal cells that lie just above them, certainly form a pluripotential reserve cell that, unlike the surrounding epithelium, usually survives injury (Boers et al., 1998; Adamson & Bowden, 1979; Evans et al., 1976). Procedures that involve denuding the trachea have demonstrated the capacity of basal cells to produce all the major cell phenotypes found in the trachea, including basal, ciliated, globet and granular secretory cells (Inamaya et al., 1989 & 1988; Liu et al., 2004 & 1994).

Lung cancer results from complex, genetic and epigenetic changes characterized by stepwise malignant progression of cancer cells in association with accumulations of genetic alterations (Fong et al., 1995; Nettesheim et al., 1990). This process, referred to as multi-step carcinogenesis, develops through the clonal evolution of initiated lung cells. Initiation consists of the acquisition of defined genetic alterations in a small number of genes that confer a proliferative advantage that facilitates progression towards invasive neoplasia. Although many of these genetic changes occur independently of histological type, their frequency and timing of occurrence with respect to cancer progression is different in small lung carcinomas (SCLC) that may originate from epithelial cells with neuro-endocrine features, and non-small cell lung carcinomas (NSCLC), they originate from bronchial, bronchiolar or alveolar epithelial cells. Furthermore, a number of genetic and epigenetic differences have been identified between squamous cell carcinoma (SCC) that arises from bronchial epithelial cells through a squamous metaplasia/displasia process and adenocarcinoma (ADC) that derives from alveolar or bronchiolar epithelial cells.

3.3.2. Squamous Cell Carcinoma of the Lung

The changes in tumorigenesis in human squamous cell carcinoma of the lung are progressive and can be described as six histologically defined stages. From the earliest to the most advanced, these stages include hyperplasia, metaplasia, progressive dysplasia, carcinoma in situ, invasive cancer, and metastatic cancer (Petersen & Petersen, 2001).

The stem cell for the squamous epithelium of the proximal airways is not certain, but is presumed that the basal cells represent a relatively quiescent zone that is the precursor. The squamous cell carcinoma, from which diagnostic criteria include evidence of squamous differentiation such as keratin formation, also show over-expression of p63, a p53-related isoform gene essential for the formation of squamous epithelia, as has been observed (Figure 3).

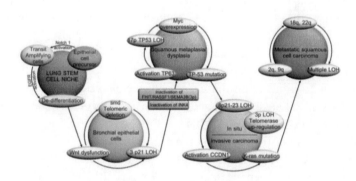

Figure 3. Proposed model for the development of squamous cell carcinoma of the lung (SCC), implicated stem cell and genetic changes.

The cell origin is believed to be a pluripotential bronchial reserve cells. It has been proposed that ADC according to their central (bronchial) or peripheral (alveolar parenchyma) location arises from two distant cells, bronchial epithelial and Clara cell type, respectively, with different mutational patterns. Since most adenocarcinomas have mixed patterns combining both central (acinar, solid) and peripheral (bronchio-alveolar, papillary) adenocarcinoma patterns, it is likely they originate, like adenosquamous carcinoma, from a common intermediate bronchial-Clara type II cell (Figure 4).

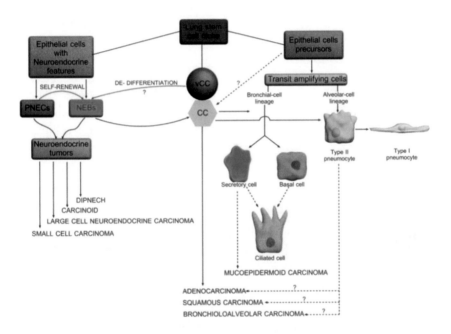

Figure 4. Developmental proposed model that implicates the different lung tumor genesis from proliferative cell types described in conducting airways. PNECs: pulmonary neuroendocrine cells. NEBs: neuroepithelial bodies. DIPNECH: diffuse idiopathic pulmonary neuroendocrine cell hyperplasia. vCC: variant clara cell.

3.3.3. Stem Cells and Oral Cancer

Like many epithelial tumors, head and neck squamous cell carcinoma (HNSCC) contains a heterogeneous population of cancer cells, some of which is accounted for by ongoing mutation that occurs because of genetic instability and environmental factors (Jain et al., 2004). The tumors demonstrate cytological and architectural features similar to normal squamous epithelium, including differentiation from a basal layer toward an apical layer containing cells with mature squamous morphology and the formation of keratin pearls.

Evidence for a developmental hierarchy in HNSCC comes from the histology and IHC studies done on moderately to well differentiated tumors. Well-to moderately-differentiated HNSCC demonstrates a cellular organization with differentiation from a basal layer with cells of immature morphology toward an apical layer with a more mature-appearing squamous morphology. By immunohistochemical analysis (IHC), performed to determine the physical location of the tumorigenic population of cells within the tumor, demonstrated that CD44+ cells expression is detected in the basal layer but not in the differentiated cells. Thus, the basal cell layer represents the undifferentiated cells, and contain with Cytokeratin 5/14 (CK5/14), a marker of normal squamous epithelial stem and progenitor cells (Chu & Weiss, 2002). Involucrin, a differentiated keratinocyte marker (Walts et al., 1985), stains the regions of the tumor that are negative for CD44+ (Prince & Ailles, 2008 & 2007). These findings provide further evidence that HNSCC is organized into a developmental hierarchy, as is predicted by the Cancer stem cell (CSC) theory of carcinogenesis.

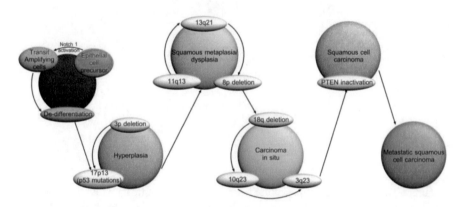

Figure 5. Proposed model for the development of squamous cell carcinoma of the oral mucosa, implicated stem cell and genetic changes.

Hypothesis concerning the origin of oral cancer stem cells (Costea et al., 2006) is as follows: 1) multiple genetic changes leading normal epithelium stem cells to transform into CSC, 2) *cell fusion* between an hematopoietic stem cell and a mutated oral keratinocyte could occur, thus leading to genetic instability, aneuplody and a cell with an altered genome that is equal to a cancer stem cell; 3) oncogenic events could occur initially in a transit amplifying (TA) cell delaying differentiation and permitting acquisition of additional oncogenic events (*de-differentiation*) leading to cancer transformation; and 4) exposure of cells to genotoxic agents could alter the cellular genomic pattern (*neosis*), resulting in the formation of epithelial cells with CSC properties (Figure 5).

3.3.4. Squamous Cell Carcinoma of the Head and Neck

The development of HNSCC is a multi-step process that involves changes related to specific genes, epigenetic events, and signal transduction within the cell. Reports indicate that of these new cases, approximately 90% of oral malignancies involving the oral cavity or adjacent structures are carcinomas.

Oral mucosal squamous cell originates in the basal cell layer of the oral mucosa. The typical presentation for an oral mucosal squamous cell carcinoma is most commonly a symptomatic or asymptomatic superficial ulcer. These superficial ulcers often progress into a symptomatic or asymptomatic exophytic nodule or tumor with an eroded/ulcerated surface. Most oral mucosal squamous cell carcinomas begin as superficial ulcerations progressing to direct invasion of the deeper structures in a firm, non-movable mass.

The high-risk of oral carcinoma are the floor of the mouth, the ventrolateral tongue, the lingual aspect of the retromolar trigone, the palate, and the anterior tonsillar pillar.

Oral leukoplakia, characterized by whitish mucosal plaques, is the most common identifiable precursor of HNSCC. Patients who present with leukoplakia followed for a mean of 8 years demonstrated a 24% risk for progression to HNSCC. Leukoplakia and Erythroplakia, which is less prevalent but has a higher risk for progression to cancer, comprise the category of oral intraepithelial neoplasia. Erythroplakia can appear as an innocuous lesion that is asymptomatic. The lesion is red in color, inflammatory, and atrophic. Erythroplakia is a common presentation of oral cavity cancers, especially in patients who smoke and drink.

Leukoplakia is a whitish mucosal lesion that does not rub off and is not associated with any disease process. It is rarely pre-cancerous. Only about 6% of early invasive carcinomas or carcinomas in situ have been shown to be purely white lesions.

3.4. Stem Cell Signaling Pathways

By definition, both normal and CSCs must maintain a self-renewal capacity in addition to giving rise to differentiated progeny cells, and thus there is likely to be similarly in the pathways governing these processes between normal and CSCs. Understanding the signaling pathways and the molecular mechanisms that are responsible for regulating these events in CSCs is extremely important, as it is likely that tumor growth is determined in part by disregulation of the Hh, Wnt, Notch and other signaling pathways (Lobo et al., 2007).

Hedgehog Signaling Pathway

The Hh gene family encodes several secreted glycoproteins such as Indian Hedgehog (Ihh), Desert Hedgehog (Dhh), and Sonic Hedgehog (Shh). These serve to mediating signaling in embryogenesis and development through activation of the Gli family transcription factors (reviewed in Taipale & Beachy, 2001; Liu et al., 2005). The Hh pathway is somewhat unique in that the signals serve to relieve a series of repressive interactions. The receptor for Hh, the transmembrane protein, Patched 1 (Ptch), normally binds and inhibits smoothened (Smoh), a G-protein-coupled receptor that is related to Fz. When secreted Hh binds both Ptch and Hedgehog-interactin protein (Hip), Smoh initiates a transcriptional response. Specifically, Smoh activates the serine/threonine kinase Fused (Fu) to release Gli from the sequestration by Suppressor of Fused (SuFu). Subsequently, Gli proteins are able to translocate to the nucleus and regulate transcription of cyclin D and E, c-myc, and other genes involved in cell proliferation and differentiation (reviewed in Nybakken & Perrimon, 2002; Pasca di Magliano & Hebrok, 2003).

Wnt Signaling Pathway

Wnts are a 19-member family of secreted glycoproteins that bind to several different cell surface receptors and determine signal transduction by the canonical or non-canonical pathway (Cadigan & Nusse, 1997). Wnt binding to LRP 5/6 and Frizzled receptors on a Dishevelled (Dvl) platform inhibits GSK-3β, which, in absence of Wnt binding, is found in complexes with axin and APC and phosphorylates β-catenin, marking it for proteolytic degradation. The accumulation of free β-catenin in the cytoplasm and nucleus is followed by direct association with the transcription factors TCF/LEF, resulting in subsequent activation of Wnt target genes that involve epithelia-to-mesenchymal transition (EMT) and cell proliferation (e.g. c-myc, cyclcin D1 , and CD44).

Wnt/β-catenin pathway is important for cell proliferation, differentiation, and self-renewal in hematopoietic stem cells (reviewed in Mohinta et al., 2007). In addition, defects in Wnt signaling are associated with several tumor types including colon, skin, breast, prostate and lung cancer (Taipale & Beachy, 2001; Reya et al., 2003; Bastian et al., 2006; Mohinta et al., 2007; Bruxvoort et al., 2007).

Notch Signaling Pathway

The Notch family transmembrane receptors is comprised of 4 members in mammals (Notch1 to Notch4) (Fleming, 1998). The mammalian Notch receptors (Notch1-Notch4) are activated by five ligands (Jagged1 and Jagged2, homologs of Serrate; and Delta1, Delta3 and Delta4, homologs of Delta). The common structural feature of Notch ligands is an N-terminal domain, DSL (Delta, Serrate and Lag).

The extracellular domains of Notch receptors contain EGF-like repeats (36 in Notch, Notch1 and Notch2; 34 in Notch3, 29 in Notch4) associated with ligand binding and three cysteine-rich Notch/LIN12 repeats (LIN) that prevent ligand-independent signaling. The cytoplasmic portion contains two protein-protein interaction domains, the RAM domain (r), six ankryin (ANK) repeats, two nuclear localization signals (NLS), a transactivation domain (TAD, absent from Notch3 and Notch4) and a PEST sequence (P).

Notch signaling often controls binary cell-fate decisions between cells that are initially equivalent with respect to their development potential (Artavanis-Tsakonas et al., 1999). Importantly, although such binary cell fate choices are classicaly associated with Notch signaling, the pathway is also widely used in patterning interactions that occur between all types that are initially distinct from one another, termed inductive cell fate interactions. Accordingly, Notch signaling depends upon direct contact between the interacting cells.

Given the wide-ranging importance of Notch signaling during animal development, it is not surprising that mutations in genes encoding Notch signaling components have been implicated in several human diseases involving aberrant cellular differentiation or tissue development.

Depending on the tumor type, Notch can variously promote or limit tumor growth through either cell autonomous or cell non-autonomous effects on differentiation, cellular metabolism, cell cycle progression, angiogenesis, and possibly self-renewal and immune function. Aberrant Notch signaling is necessary not only for the initiation of tumors but also for tumor maintenance

(Weng et al., 2003; Roy et al., 2007). The effects of Notch on individual cells are highly dependent on signal dose and context. In cancer, Notch can variously serve as an oncogen or a tumor suppressor, a repressor or inducer of terminal differentiation, and perhaps a cancer stem cell factor in specific contexts.

The clearest example of oncogenic Notch signaling is found in T-acute lymphoblastic leukemia/lymphoma (T-ALL) through Notch1 involvement (van Vlierberghe et al., 2006; Chiang et al., 2006). Other data suggests that Notch1 also suppresses p53 function in T-ALL cells (Beverly et al., 2005) which could promote oncogenesis through increased cell survival and genomic inestability.

Notch signals are oncogenic in breast and salivary gland epithelium (Jhappan et al., 1992). The expression of Notch receptors is increased in the human breast (Weijzen et al., 2002; Reedijk et al., 2005), and the expression of ligands such as Jagged1, correlates with a more aggressive disease course in both breast and prostate cancer (Reedijk et al., 2005; Santagata et al., 2004; Bismar et al., 2006). The expression of Notch receptors and their downstream target genes is also upregulated in primary human melanomas (Balint et al., 2005; Hoek et al., 2004), and enforced expression of constitutively active Notch1 promotes melanoma progression (Balint et al., 2005; Liu et al., 2006). Other neoplasias have implicated Notch in their pathogenesis, such as medulloblastoma (Marino, 2005; Hallahan et al., 2004) and ovarian cancer (Park et al., 2006).

In some contexts, Notch is a tumor suppressor. Notch has important roles in normal arteriogenesis and neo-angiogenesis, both of which are likely to be recapitulated in cancers (Rehman & Wang, 2006). In some instances, Notch signaling in endothelial cells appears to be triggered by ligands expressed on tumor cells (Zeng et al., 2005), which might contribute to the aggresive clinical behavior of tumors expressing high levels of Notch ligands (Reedijk et al., 2005; Santagata et al., 2004; Bismar et al., 2006).

The molecular mechanisms by which aberrant Notch signaling causes cancer are not fully understood. Experimentally, Notch1 can collaborate with c-myc (Girad et al., 1996; Palomero et al., 2006; Sharma et al., 2006), E2A-PBX1 (Rohn et al., 1996) and Ikaros (Beverly & Capobianco, 2003), whereas Notch3 downregulates tumor suppressive E2A activity (Talora et al., 2003). Notch1 inhibits p53-mediated apoptosis by stimulating signaling through the PI3K-Akt-mTOR-eIF4E pathway (Mungamuri et al., 2006), and antagonizes the growth suppressive effects of the transforming growth factor beta (TGF-β) signaling pathways (Sun et al., 2005). Other researchers suggest the existence of an intimate and functionally important interaction between Notch and hypoxia-inducible factor (HIF)-1α , a transcription factor that regulates many genes involved in the response to hypoxia, including factors that promote angiogenesis (Gordan & Simon, 2007). Other data suggests that HIF-1α binds and stabilizes activated Notch1, leading to enhanced Notch signaling (Gustafson et al., 2005). Expression of HIF-1α and Notch1 are correlated in breast cancer, in which Notch1 appears to upregulate HIF-1α expression (Soares et al., 2004). It is also possible that Notch ligands on tumor cells impact the host immune response through effects on B an T cells (Dallman et al., 2005).

ACKNOWLEDGEMENT

Silvia Díaz Prado is supported by an Isidro Parga Pondal contract from Xunta de Galicia, A Coruña (Spain).

REFERENCES

Abelev GI. In *Clinical Oncohematology* (Volkova, M. A., ed.) [in Russian], 2nd Edn., Meditsina, Moscow, 2007, pp.167-176.

Adamson IY, Bowden DH. Bleomycin-induced injury and metaplasia of alveolar type 2 cells. Relationship of cellular responses to drug presence in the lung. *Am J pathol* 1979;96:531-544.

Anton Aparicio LM, Diaz Prado S. Understanding stem cells. The lung and the airway. Clinical Trans Oncol. *Invited Monograph* 2007/1.

Aparicio Gallego G, Diaz Prado S, Garcia Campleo R, Alonso Curbera G. The airways stem cells. In: Understanding stem cells. The lung and the airway. *Clin Trans Oncol. Invited Monography* 2007/1:24-33.

Artavanis-Tsakonas S, Rand MD, Lake RJ. Notch signaling; cell fate control and signal integration in development. *Science* 1999; 284:770-6.

Auerbach O, Forman JB, Gere JB, Kassouny DY, Muehsam GE, Petrick TG, Smolin HJ, Stout AP. Changes in the bronchial epithelium in relation to smoking and cancer of the lung. *N Engl J Med* 1957;256:98-104.

Auerbach O, Hammond EC, Garfinkel L. Changes in bronchial epithelium in relation to cigarette smoking, 1955-1960 vs 1970-1977. *N Engl J Med* 1979;300:381-5.

Auerbach S, Stout AP, Hammond EC,Garfinkel L. Changes in bronchial epithelium in relation to cigarette smoking and in relation to lung cancer. *N Engl J Med* 1961;265:253-267.

Balint K, Xiao M, Pinnix CC, Soma A, Veres I, Juhasz I, Brown EJ, Capobianco AJ, Herlyn M, Liu ZJ. Activation of Notch1 signaling is required for β-catenin-mediated human primary melanoma progression. *J Clin Invest* 2005;115:3166-3176.

Bastian PJ, Ellinger J, Wellmann A, Wernert N, Heukamp LC, Muller SC, von Ruwcker A. Diagnostic and information in prostate cancer with the help of a small set of hypermethylated gene loci. *Clin Cancer Res* 2006;11:4097-4106.

Berenblum I, Shubick P. The role of croton oil applications, associated with a single painting of a carcinogen, in tumor induction of the mouse's skin. *Br J cancer* 1947; 1:379-382.

Beverly LJ, Capobianco AJ. Perturbation of Ikaros isoform selection by MLV integration is a cooperative event in Notch(IC)-induced T cell leukemogenesis. *Cancer Cell* 2003:3:551-564.

Beverly LJ, Felsher DW, Capobianco AJ. Suppression of p53 by Notch in lymphomagenesis: implications for initiation and regression. *Cancer Res* 2005;65:7159-7168.

Bishop AE. Pulmonary epithelial stem cells. *Cell Prolif* 2003;37:89-96.

Bismar TA, Demichelis F, Riva A, Kim R, Varambally S, He L, Kutok J, Aster JC, Tang J, Kuefer R, Hofer MD, Febbo PG, Chinnaiyan AM, Rubin MA. Defining aggressive prostate cancer using a 12-gene model. *Neoplasia* 2006; 8:59-68.

Boers JE, Ambergen AW, Thunnissen FB. Number and proliferation of basal and parabasal cells in normal airway epithelium. *Am J Respir Crit Care Med* 1998;157:2000-2006.

Braakhuis BJ, Leemans CR, Brakenhoff RH. Expanding fields of genetically-altered cells in head and neck squamous carcinogenesis. *Semin Cancer Biol* 2005;15:113-120.

Braakhuis BJ, Tabor MP, Kummer JA , Leemans CR, Brakenhoff RH. A genetic explanatioin of Slaughter's concept of field cancerization: evidence and clinical implications. *Cancer Res* 2003;63:1727-1730.

Brennan JA, Mao L, Hruban RH, Boyle JO, Eby YJ, Koch WM, Goodman SN, Sidransky D. Molecular assessment of histopathological staging in squamous cell carcinoma of the head and neck. *N Engl J Med* 1995;332:429-435.

Bruxvoort KJ, Charbonneau HM, Giambernardi TA, Goolsby JC, Qian CN, Zylstra CR, Robinson DR, Roy-BurmanP, Shaw AK, Buckner-Berghuis BD, Singler RE, Resau JH, Sillivan R, Busjman W, Williams BO. Inactivation of Apc in the mouse prostate causes prostate carcinoma. *Cancer Res* 2007;67:2490-2496.

Cadigan KM, Nusse R. Wnt signaling: a common theme in animal development. *Genes Dev* 1997;11:3286-3305.

Califano J, Leong PL, Koch WM, Eisenberger CF, Sidransky D, Westra WH. Second esophageal tumors in patients with head and neck squamous cell carcinoma: an assessment of clonal relationship. *Clin Cancer Res* 1999;5:1862-1867.

Chan EF, Gat U McNiff JM, Fuchs E. A common human skin tumor is caused by activation mutations in beta-catenin. *Nat Genet* 1999;21(4):410-413.

Chiang MY, Xu ML, Histen G, Shestova O, Roy M, Nam Y, Blacklow SC, Sacks DB, Pear WS, Aster JC. Identification of a conserved negative regulatory sequence that influences the leukemogenic activity of NOTCH1. *Mol Cell Biol* 2006;26;6261-6271.

Chu PG, Weiss LM. Keratin expression in human tissues and neoplasms. *Histopathology* 2002;40:403-39.

Chung LW, Baseman A, Assikis V, Zhau HE. Molecular insights into prostate cancer progression: the missing link of tumor micro-environment. *J Urol* 2005;173:10-20.

Clarke MF. A self-renewal assay for cancer stem cells. *Cancer Chemother Pharmacol* 2005; 56 suppl 1:64-68.

Costea DE, Tsinkalovsky O, Vintermyr OK, Johannessen AC, Mackenzie IC. Cancer stem cells- new and potentially important targets for the therapy of oral squamous cell carcinoma. *Oral Dis* 2006;12:443-454.

Dallman MJ, Smith E, Benson RA, Lamb JR. Notch: control of lymphocyte differentiation in the periphery. *Curr Opin Immunol* 2005;17:259-266.

Emura E. Stem cells of the respiratory tract. *Paed Respir Rev* 2002;3:36.

Emura E. Stem cells on the respiratory epithelium and their in vitro cultivation. *Cell Dev Biol Anim* 1997;33:3-14.

Evans MJ, Johnson LV, Stephens RJ, Freman G. Renewal of the terminal bronchiolar epithelium in the rat following exposure to NO_2 or O_3 . *Lab Invest* 1976;35:246-257.

Fidler IJ, Talmadge JE. Evidence that intravenously derived murine pulmonary melanoma metastases can originate from the expansion of a single tumor cell. *Cancer Res* 1986; 46:5167-71.

Fleishman EV. In *Clinical Oncohematology* (Volkova, M. A, ed.) [in Russian], 2nd Edn., Meditsina, Moscow, 2007, pp. 370-408.

Fleming RJ. Structural conservation of Notch receptors and ligands. *Semin Cell Dev Biol* 1998;9:599-607.

Fong KM, Zimmerman PV, Smith PJ. Lung pathology: The molecular genetics of non-small cell lung cancer. *Pathology* 1995;27:295-301.

Forastiere A, Koch W, Trotti A, Sidransky D. Medical progress-head and neck cancer. *New Engl J Med* 2001;345:1890-1900.

Freeman E. Periodontium. In: *Oral Histology: Development Structure and Functions*. Ten Cate AR ed. Mosby, St Louis 1998;pp:253-288.

Friedwald WF, Rous P. The initiation and promoting elements in tumor production. An analysis of the effects of tar, benzopyrene and methylcholantrene on rabbit skin. *J Exp Med* 1944;80:1001-126.

Fuchs E. Das Sarkom des Uvealtractus. *Graefe's Arch Ophthalmol* 1882;XII,233.

Gazdar AF, Linnaoila TR, Foley JF. Peripheral airway cell differentiation in human lung cancer cell lines. *Cancer Res* 1990;50:5481-5487.

Ghazizadeh S, Taichman LB. Organization of stem cells and their progeny in human epidermis. *Invest Dermatol* 2005;124:367-372.

Giangreco A, Reynolds SD, Stripp BR. Terminal bronchioles harbor a unique airway stem cell population that localizes to the bronchioalveolar junction. *Am J Pathol* 2002;161:173-182.

Girad L, Hanna Z, Beaulieu N, Hoemann CD, Simard C, Kozak CA, Jolicoeur P. Frequent pro-virus insertional mutagenesis of Notch1 in thymomas of MMTVD/myc transgenic mice suggests a collaboration of c-myc and Notch 1 for oncogenesis. *Genes Dev* 1996;10:1930-1944.

Gordan JD, Simon MC. Hypoxia-inducible factors: central regulators of the tumor phenotype. *Curr Opin Genet Dev* 2007; 17:71-77.

Gronthos S, Brahim J, Li W, Fisher LW, Cherman N, Boyde A, DenBesten P, Robey PG, Shi A. Stem cell properties of human dental pulp stem cells. *J Dent Res* 2002;81:531-535.

Gronthos S, Mankani M, Brahim J, Robey PG, Shi S. Postnatal human dental pulp stem cells (DPSCs) in vitro and in vivo. *Proc Natl Acad Sci USA* 2000;97:13625-13630.

Gustafsson MV, Zheng X, Pereira T, Gradin K, Jin S. Lundkvist J, Ruas JL, Poellinger L, Lendahl U, Bondeson M. Hypoxia requires notch signaling to maintain the undifferentiated cell state. *Dev Cell* 2005;9:617-628.

Hakeyama S, Yaegashi T, Takeda Y, Kurimatsu K. Localization of bromodeoxyuridine-incorporating, p63- and p75^{NGFR} expressing cells in the human gingival epithelium. *J Oral Science* 2007;49:287-291.

Hallahan AR, Pritchard JI, Hansen S, Benson M, Stoeck J, Hatton BA, Russell TL, Ellenbogen RG, Bernstein ID, Beachy PA, Olson JM. The SmoA1 mouse model reveals that Notch signaling is critical for the growth and survival of sonic hedgehog-induced medulloblastomas. *Cancer Res* 2004; 64:7794-7800.

Hanahan D, Weinberg RA. The hallmarks of cancer. *Cell* 2000; 100:57-70.

Harada H, Kettunen P, Jung HS, Mustonen T, Wang YA, Thesleff I. Localization of putative stem cells in dental epithelium and their association with Notch and FGF signaling. *J Cell Biol* 1999;147:105-120.

Hatakeyama S, Yaegashi T, Oikawa Y, Fujiwara H, Mikami T, Takeda Y, Satoh M. Expression pattern of adhesion molecules in junctional epithelium differs from that in other gingival epithelia. *J Periodont Res* 2006;41:322-328.

Hewitt RE, McMarlin A, Kleiner D, Wersto R, Martin P, Tsokos M, Stamp GW, Stetler-Stevenson WG. Validation of a model of colon cancer progression. *J Pathol* 2000;192:446-454.

Hoek K, Rimm DL, Williams KR, Zhao H, Ariyan G, Lin A, Kluger HM, Berger AJ, Cheng E, Trombetta ES, Wu T, Niinobe M, Yoshikawa K, Hannigan GE, Halaban R. Expression profiling reveals novel pathways in the transformation of melanocytes to melanoma. *Cancer Res* 2004;64:5270-5282.

Huntly BJ, Gilliland DG. Leukemia stem cells and the evolution of cancer-stem-cell research. *Nat Rev Cancer* 2005;5:311-321.

Inamaya Y, Hook GE, Brody AR, Cameron GS, Jetten AM, Gilmore LB, Gray T, Nettesheim P. The differentiation potential of tracheal basal cells. *Lab Invest* 1988;58:706-717.

Inamaya Y, Hook GE, Brody AR, Jetten AM, Gray T, Mahler J, Nettesheim P. In vitro and in vivo growth and differentiation of clones of tracheal basal cells. *Am J Pathol* 1989;134:539-549.

Jain S, Khuri FR, Shin DM. Prevention of head and neck cancer: current status and future prospects. *Curr Probl Cancer* 2004;28:265-86.

Jhappan C, Gallahan D, Stahle C, Chu E, Smith GH, Merlino G, Callahan R. Expression of an activated Notch-related int-3 transgene interferes with cell differentiation and induces neoplastic transformation in mammary and salivary glands. *Genes Dev* 1992; 6:345-55.

Jordan CT. Cancer stem cell biology: from leukemia to solid tumors. *Curr Opin Cell Biol* 2004;16:708-712.

Kennaway E. Identification of a carcinogenic compound in coal tar. *Br Med J* 1955;2:749-752.

Kettunen P, Karavanoma I, Thesleff I. Responsiveness of developing dental tissues to fibroblast growth factors: expression of splicing alternatives of FGFR1, -2, -3, and of FGFR4; and stimulation of cell proliferation by FGF-2, -4, -8, and -9. *Dev Genet* 1998;22:374-385.

Klein OD, Lyons DB, Balooch G, Marshall GW, Basson MA, Peterka M, Boran T, Peterkova R, Martin GR. An FGF-signaling loop sustains the generation of differentiated progeny from stem cells in mouse incisors. *Development* 2008;135:377-385.

Langley RR, Fidler IJ. Tumor cell-organ micro-environment interactions in the pathogenesis of cancer metastasis. *Endocr Rev* 2007;28:297-321.

Lengauer C, Kinzler KW, Vogelstein B. Genetic insatilities in human cancers. *Nature* 1998;396:643-649.

Li A, Simmons PJ, Kam P. Identification and isolation of candidate human keratinocyte stem cells based on cell surface phenotype. *Proc Natl Acad Sci USA* 1998;95:3902-3903.

Liu ZJ, Xiao M, Balint K, Smalley KS, Brafford P, Qiu R, Pinnix CC, Li X, Herlyn M. Notch1 signaling promotes primary melanoma progression by activating mitogen-activated protein kinase/phosphatidylinositol 3-kinase-Akt pathways and up-regulating N-cadherin expression. *Cancer Res* 2006;66:4182-4190.

Liu JY, Natteshein P, Raandalll SH. Growth and differentiation of tracheal progenitor cells. *Am J Physiol* 1994;266:L296-307.

Liu S, Dontu G, Wicha MA. Mammary stem cells, self-renewal pathways, and carcinogenesis. *Breast Cancer Res* 2005;7:86-95.

Liu X, Driskel RR, Engelhardt JF. Airway glandular development and stem cells. *Curr Top Dev Biol* 2004;64:33-56.

Lobo NA, Shimono Y, Qian D, Clarke MF. The biology of cancer stem cells. *Annu Rev Cell Dev Biol* 2007;23:675-699.

Mackenzie IC. Growth of malignant oral epithelial stem cells after seeding into organotypical cultures of normal mucosa. *J Oral Pathol Med* 2004;33:71-78.

Marino S. Medulloblastoma: development mechanisms out of control. *Trends Mol Med* 2005;11:17-22.

Mohinta S, Wu H, Chaurasia P, Watabe K. Wnt pathway and breast cancer. *Front Biosci* 2007;12:4020-4033.

Moolgavkar SH, Luebeck EG. Multi-stage carcinogenesis and the incidence of human cancer. *Genes Chromosomes Cancer* 2003;38:302-306.

Müller A, Homey B, Soto H, Ge N, Catron D, Buchanan ME, McClanahan T, Murphy E, Yuan W, Wagner SN, Barrera JL, Mohar A, Verástegui E, Zlotnik A. Involvement of chemokine receptors in breast cancer metastasis. *Nature* 2001;410:50-56.

Mungamuri SK, Yang X, Thor AD, Somasundaram K. Survival-signaling by Notch1: mammalian target of rapamycin (mTOR)-dependent inhibition of p53. *Cancer Res* 2006;66:4715-4724.

Murphy PM. Chemokines and the molecular basis of cancer metastasis. *N Engl J Med* 2001;345:833-835.

Nettesheim P, Jetten AM, Inamaya Y, Brody AR, George MA, Gilmore LB, Gray T, Hook GE. Pathways of differentiation of airway epithelial cells. *Environ Health Perspect* 1990; 85:317-29.

Nybakken K, Perrimon N. Hedgehog signal transduction: recent findings . *Curr Opin Genet Dev* 2002;12:503-511.

Owens DM, Watt FM. Contribution of stem cells and differentiated cells to epidermal tumors. *Nat Rev Cancer* 2003;3:444-451.

Paget S. The distribution of secondary growths in cancer of the breast. *Lancet* 1889;133;571-573.

Palomero T, Lim WK, Odom DT, Sulis ML, Real PJ, Margolin A, Barnes KC, O'Neil J, Neuberg D, Weng AP, Aster JC, Sigaux F, Soulier J, Look AT, Young RA, Califano A, Ferrando AA. Notch1 directly regulates c-MYC and activates as feed-forward-loop transcriptional network promoting leukemic cell growth. *Proc Natl Acad Sci USA* 2006;103:18261-18266.

Pardal R, Clarke MF, Morrison SJ. Applying the principles of stem cell biology to cancer. *Nat Rev Cancer* 2003;3:895-902.

Park JY, Li M, Nakayama K, Mao TL, Davidson B, Zhang Z, Kurman RJ, Eberhart CG, Shih I, Wang TL. Notch3 gene amplification in ovarian cancer. *Cancer Res* 2006;66:6312-6318.

Pasca di Magliano M, Hebrok M. Hedgehog signaling in cancer formation and maintenance. *Nat Rev Cancer* 2003; 3:903-11.

Perez-Losada J, Balmain A. Stem-cell hierarchy in skin cancer. *Nat Rev Cancer* 2003;3:434-443.

Perryman SV, Sylvester KG. Repair and regeneration: opportunities for carcinogenesis from tissue stem cells. *J Cell Mol Med* 2006;10:292-308.

Petersen I, Petersen S. Towards a genetic-based classification on human lung cancer. *Anal Cell Pathol* 2001;22:111-121.

Prince M, Ailles LE. Cancer stem cells in head and neck squamous cell cancer. *J Clin Oncol* 2008;26:2871-2875.

Prince M, Sivanandan R, Kaczorowski A, Wolf GT, Kaplan MJ, Dalerba P, Weissman IL, Clarke MF, Ailles LE. Identification of a subpopulation of cell with cancer stem cell properties in head and neck squamous cell carcinoma. *Poc Natl Acad Sci USA* 2007;104:973-978.

Rajagopalan H, Nowak MA, Vogelstein B, Lengauer C. The significance of unstable chromosomes in colorectal cancer. *Nat Rev Cancer* 2003;3:695-701.

Reedijk M, Odoric S, Chang L, Zhang H, Miller N, McCready DR, Lockwood G, Egan SE. High-level coexpression of JAG1 and NOTCH1 is observed in human breast cancer and is associated with poor overall survival. *Cancer Res* 2005;65:8530-8537.

Rehman AO, Wang CY. Notch signaling in the regulation of tumor angiogenesis. *Trends Cell Biol* 2006;16:293-300.

Reya T, Duncan AW, Ailles L, Domen J, Scherer DC, Willert K, Hintz L, Nusse R, Weissman IL. A role for Wnt signaling in self-renewal of hematopoietic stem cells. *Nature* 2003;423:409-414.

Rohn JL, Lauring AS, Linenberg MI, Overbaugh J. Transduction of Notch2 in feline leukemia virus-induced thymic lymphoma. *J Virol* 1996;70:8071-8880.

Rous P, Kidd JG. Conditional neoplasms and subthreshold neoplastic states. A study of the tar tumors of rabbits. *J Exp Med* 1942;73:365-390.

Roy M, Pear WS, Aster JC. The multi-faceted role of Notch in cancer. *Curr Opin Gene Dev* 2007;17:52-59.

Santagata S, Demichelis F, Riva A, Varambally S, Hofer MD, Kutoh JL, Kim R, Tang J, Montie JE, Chinnaiyan AM, Rubin MA, Aster JC. JAGGED1 expression is associated with prostate cancer metastasis and recurrence. *Cancer Res* 2004;64:6854-6857.

Sharma VM, Calvo JA, Drahein KM, Cunninham LA, Hermance N, Beverly L, Krishnamoorthy V, Bhasin M, Capobianco AJ, Kelliher MA. Notch1 contributes to mouse T-cell leukemia by directly inducing the expression of c-myc. *Mol Cell Biol* 2006;26:8022-8031.

Slaugther DP; Saothwick HW, Smejkal W. Field cancerization in oral stratified squamous epithelium. *Cancer* 1953;6:963-968.

Soares R, Balogh G, Guo S, Gartner F, Russo J, Schmitt F. Evidence for the notch signaling pathway on the role of estrogen in angiogenesis. *Mol Endocrinol* 2004;18:2333-2343.

Stetler-Stevenson WG. The role of matrix metalloproteinases in tumor invasion, metastasis, and angiogenesis. *Surg Oncol Clin North Am* 2001;10:383-392.

Stingl J, Caldas C. Molecular heterogenicity of breast carcinomas and the cancer stem cell hypothesis. *Nat Rev Cancer*. 2007;7:791-799.

Strieter RM. Chemokines: not just leukocyte chemoattractans in the promotion of cancer. *Nat Immunol* 2001;2:285-286.

Sun Y, Lowther W, Kato K, Blanco C, Kenney N, Strizzi KL, Raafat D, Hirota M, Khan NI, Bargo S, Jones B, Salomon D, Callahan R. Notch4 intracellular domain binding to Smad3 and inhibition of the TGF-β signaling. *Oncogene* 2005;24:5365-5374.

Tabor MP, Brakenhoff RH, van Houten VM, Kummer JA, Snel MH, Snijders PJ, Snow GB, Leemans CR, Braakhuis BJ. Persistence of genetically altered fields in head and neck cancer patients:biological and clinical implications. *Clin Cancer Res* 2001;7:1523-1532.

Taipale J, Beachy PA. The Hedgehog and Wnt signaling pathways in cancer. *Nature* 2001;411:349-354.

Talora C, Campese AF, Bellavia D, Pascucci M, Checquolo S, Groppioni M, Frati L, von Boehmer H, Gulino A, Screpanti I. Pre-TCR-triggered ERK signaling-dependent downregulation of E2A activivty. *EMBO Rep* 2003;4:1067-1072.

Tang DG, Patrawala L, Calhoun T, Bathia B, Choy G, Schnneider-Broussard R, Jeter C. Prostate cancer stem/progenitor cells: Identification , characterization and implications. *Mol Carcinog* 2007;46:1-14.

Tatosyan AG. In *Carcinogenesis* (Zaridze, D. G., ed.) [in Russian], Meditsina, Moscow, 2004, pp. 103-124.

Tummers M, Thesleff I. Toot or crown: a developmental choice orchestrated by the differential regulation of the epithelial stem cell niche in the tooth of two rodent species. *Development* 2003;130:1049-1057.

Van Vlierberghe P, Meijerink JP, Lee C, Ferrando AA, Look AT, van Wering ER, Beverloo HB, Aster JC, Pieters R. A new recurrent 9q34 duplication in pediatric T-cell acute lymphoblastic leukemia. *Leukemia* 2006; 20:1245-1253.

Vogelstein B, Kinzler KW. The multi-step nature of cancer. Trands Genet 1993;9:138-141.

Walts AE, Said JW, Siegel MB, Banks-Schlegel S. Involucrin, a marker of squamous and urothelial differentiation. An immunohistochemical study on its distribution in normal and neoplastic tissues. *J Pathol* 1985;145:329-40.

Wang X-P, Suomalainen M, Felszeghy S, Zelarayan LC, Alonso MT, Plikus MV, Maas RL, Chuing C-M, Schimmang T, Thesleff I. An integrated gene regulatory network controls stem cell proliferation in teeth. *Biol* 2007;5:e159.

Weijzen S, Rizzo P, Braid M, Vaishnav R, Jonkheer SM, Zlobin A, Osborne BA, Gottipati S, Aster JC, Hahn WC, Rudolf M, Siziopikou K, Kast WM, Miele L. Activation of Notch-1 signaling maintain the neoplastic phenotype in human Ras-transformed cells. *Nat Med* 2002;8:979-986.

Weng AP,Nam Y, Wolfe MS, Pear WS, Griffin JD, Blacklow SC, Aster JC. Growth suppression of pre-T acute lymphoblastic leukemia cells by inhibition of notch signaling. *Mol Cell Biol* 2003;23:655-664.

Wicha MS, Liu S, Dotu G. Cancer Stem cells: and old idea a paradigm shift. *Cancer Res* 2006;66:1883-1890.

Yaamagiwa K, Ichiikawa KJ. Experimental study of the pathogenesis of cancer. *J Cancer Res* 1918;3:1-9.

Zeng Q, Li S, Chepeha DB, Giordano TJ, Li J, Zhang H, Polverini PJ, Nor J, Kitajewski J, Wang CY. Crosstalk between tumor and endothelial cells promotes tumor angiogenesis by MAPK activation of Notch signaling. *Cancer Cell* 2005;8:13-23.

Zilber LA, Irlin IS, Kiselev FL. *Evolution of the Virus-Genetic Theory of Tumor Arising*, Chap. 8, *Endogenous Viruses and "Normal" Therapy* [in Russian], Nauka, Moscow, 1975, pp. 242-310.

In: Squamous Cell Carcinoma   ISBN: 978-1-61209-929-3
Editor: Daniel V. Mortensen   © 2012 Nova Science Publishers, Inc.

Chapter 2

SQUAMOUS CELL CARCINOMA ONTOGENY: PART II

S. Díaz Prado[1,2], G. Aparicio Gallego[2], V. Medina Villaamil[2], R. García Campelo[3] and L.M. Anton Aparicio[1,3]

[1]Medicine Department. University of A Coruña, A Coruña, Spain
[2]INIBIC-Hospital Universitario A Coruña, A Coruña, Spain
[3]Medical Oncology Service. Hospital Universitario A Coruña,
A Coruña, Spain

ABSTRACT

Intermediary filaments, like cytokeratins, are essential intracellular components, underlying reflecting distinct cellular properties and differentiation stages in epithelial organs. The proteins of the cytokeratin family are epithelium specific expressed as low and high-molecular weight, acid and basic polypeptides. In general, CK expression patterns are highly-conserved. Cytokeratins (CKs) are the intermediate filament proteins of the epithelium cells which have become important markers of normal and abnormal cell differentiations. The keratin expression pattern in oral stratified epithelium is related to the cellular differentiation level: the normal pattern shows the keratin pair K5/14 in the stratum basale whereas K1/10 and k4/13, respectively, are the two pairs associated with differentiating suprabasal cells. Expression pattern of K8/18 is rather uncommon in mature squamous epithelium.

CKs alterations have been reported in carcinomas from different anatomical sites and these have been associated with specific aspects of tumor behavior.

In the literature, both quantitative and qualitative changes in catenins have been shown to be associated with dedifferentiation, dissemination of tumor cells from primary location, and prognosis in many human tumors. Yet, the exact mechanisms behind changes in the expression of catenin in cancer remains unclear. The actions of catenins in signaling pathways have only been partially clarified, but the most investigated pathway associated with catenins in humans is the so called Wnt signaling pathway. It is demonstrated that oral and lung squamous cell carcinomas express Wnt members and activate the signaling pathway. Identification of Wnt members in normal gingival keratinocytes demonstrates that head and neck carcinoma cells most frequently expressed keratinocyte-type Wnts.

Without Wnt signaling, β-catenin is readily phosphorylated and eventually degraded. The activation of the Wnt signaling pathway may block the turnover of uncomplexed β-catenin, resulting in increased cytoplasmic accumulation.

1. SQUAMOUS CELL CARCINOMA OF THE LUNG

Nearly all lung cancers exhibit the morphological and molecular features of epithelial cells, and are accordingly classified as carcinomas. The cells of origin of virtually all lung cancers reside in the epithelial lining of the airways. As more is learned about the origin of lung carcinoma, it is increasingly clear that the biology of lesions arising in the central airways is distinct from that of peripheral airway lesions. Lung carcinoma, like tumors in other organs, is thought to arise from a stepwise series of molecular and cellular alterations in precursor cells.

Lung cancers result from complex, genetic and epigenetic changes characterized by stepwise malignant progression of cancer cells in association with accumulation of genetic alterations. This process, referred to as multi-step carcinogenesis, develops through the clonal evolution of initiated lung cells. Initiation consists in the adquisition of defined genetic alterations in a small number of genes that confer a proliferative advantage that facilitates progression towards invasive neoplasia.

Although many of these genetic changes occur independently of histological type, their frequency and timing of occurrence with respect to cancer progression is different in small cell lung carcinomas (SCLC) that may originate from epithelial cells with neuro-endocrine features, and non-small cell lung carcinomas (NSCLC), they originate from bronchial, bronchiolar or alveolar epithelial cells. Furthermore, a number of genetic and epigenetic differences have been identified between squamous cell carcinoma (SCC) that arises from bronchial epithelial cells through a squamous metaplasia/dysplasia process and adenocarcinoma (ADC) that derives from alveolar or bronchiolar epithelial cells.

Lung carcinomas are usually classified as small-cell lung carcinomas (SCLC) or non-small cell lung carcinomas (NSCLC). NSCLC is histopathologically and clinically different from SCLS, and is further subcategorized as squamous cell carcinomas (SCC), adenocarcinomas (ADC), and large-cell carcinomas (LCC), of which adenocarcinomas are the most common. The changes in tumorigenesis in human squamous cell lung carcinoma are progressive and can be described as six, histologically- defined stages. From the earliest to the most advanceds, these changes include hyperplasia, metaplasia, progressive dysplasia, carcinoma in situ, invasive cancer, and metastatic cancer.

1.1. The Genetic Level

Underlying the morphological and molecular changes that occur in the airways is a multi-step sequence of events that occurs at the subcellular chromosomal levels (Table I). The initial event in lung carcinogenesis is the formation of DNA adducts, physical complexes between DNA, and the reactive metabolites in tobacco smoke and industrial pollutants (Hecht, 2002; Pfeifer et al., 2002; Wiencke, 2002).

DNA adducts activate complex DNA repair mechanisms which are not completely effective in removing adducts from damaged DNA. Unrepaired DNA bases may be bypassed by DNA polymerase, creating mutations that are transmitted to daughtther cells. Mutations formed in this way tend to favor GC→TA transversions. Many of the genetic changes that ultimately appear in lung carcinomas are thought to originally form from misrepaired DNA adducts.

Among them, the most important genetic changes are allelic losses. Chromosomal loci that normally harbor two different polymorphic alleles are assessed for the loss of one (loss of heterozygosity, LOH) or both of these alleles. Loss of both alleles (homozygous deletion) results in the slilencing of the gene while the loss of a single allele (heterozygous loss) causes loss of gene expression if the retained allele is mutated or inactivated by methylation (Girard et al., 2000; Wistuba et al., 2000 & 1999).

Table 1. Morphological and molecular changes that occur in the airways from normal epithelium to invasive carcinoma

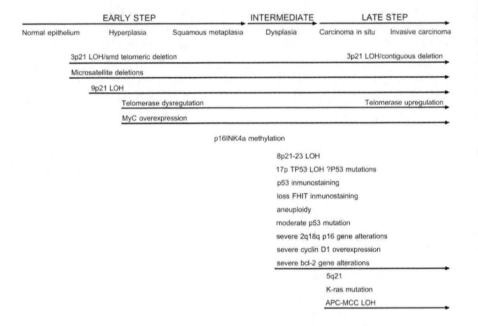

There are differences between adenocarcinoma and squamous cell carcinoma (Balsara & Testa, 2002). Squamous cell cancers have more frequent gains of 3q22-q26 and loss of 3p, when compared to adenocarcinoma (Balsara et al., 1997; Massion et al., 2002). This region of gain in squamous cell carcinoma, narrowed to a region of ~30Mb by array CGH, includes the catalytic subunit of phosphatidylinositol 3-kinase, an activator of protein kinase-B/Akt (Massion et al., 2002).

1.2. The Molecular and Cellular Level

Lung carcinoma is though to arise from a stepwise series (Vogelstein & Kinzler, 1993) of molecular and cellular alterations in the precursor cells. The cells of origin of virtually all lung cancers reside in the epithelial lining of the airways (Auerbach et al., 1962). As more is learned about the origin of lung carcinoma, it is increasingly clear that the biology of lesions arising in the central airways is distinct from that of peripheral airway lesions. In addition, there are important distinctions between tumors from the two sites in histopathological appearances.

The precursor cells, termed *central airway lesions*, are referred to tumors and pre-malignant conditions predominantly arising proximal to the terminal bronchiolar and alveolar epithelium. Typically, these lesions have been regarded as precursors of squamous carcinoma but they may also represent precursors of other histological types of central airway carcinoma.

Nearly all lung cancers exhibit the morphological and molecular features of epithelial cells and are accordingly classified as carcinomas.The classification is based on cellular changes that occur in the epithelium which consist of a transformation of bilayered mucociliary epithelium to squamous epithelium that is associated with varying degrees of alteration in nuclear irregularity and mitotic activity. The invasive cells may form keratin pearls and intercellular bridges (Travis et al., 1999) and may develop irregular areas of central necrosis described as geographic necrosis. Nuclear features include irregular nuclei and coarse chromatin. The cytoplasm may show clearing, which can resemeble vacuolization as might be seen in adenocarcinomas.

The classification includes 7 categories ranging from microscopic features including basal cell hyperplasia and squamous metaplasia that are not considered pre-malignant through mild, moderate and severe dysplasia and carcinoma *in situ* (Carter, 1985).

1.3. The Histological Level

Most cavitating lung cancers are squamous cell carcinomas, and virtually all cases show intravascular tumor cells adjacent to the tumor (Chaudhuri, 1973).

Intercellular bridging, squamous pearl formation, and individual cell keratinization characterize squamous differentiation in squamous carcinomas. In well-differentiated tumors, these features are readily apparent; however, in poorly differentiated tumors, they are difficult to find (Carlile & Edwards, 1986). Squamous tumors also elicit a variable stromal response consisting of loose fibroblastic tissue with an inflammatory component that may include plasma cells, macrophages, and lymphocytes. Histological features of SCC are summarized as chromatin coarse and clumped, nucleoli often large and misshapen, and frequent mitoses at the nucleus; abundant and eosinophilic cytoplasm; but defining features are keratin pearls, intercellular bridges, epidermoid sheets and fibrotic stromal response (Table II). Nuclear features include irregular nuclei and coarse chromatin. In more poorly differentiated carcinomas, there is less keratinization, and intercellular bridges may be difficult to identify.

Table 2. Histological features of lung squamous cell carcinoma

Subtype	Nucleus	Cytoplasm	Defining Feature(s)
Squamous (SCC)	Chromatin coarse, clumped Nucleoli often large misshapen Mitoses frequent	Abundant Eosinophilic (red)	Keratin pearls Intercelular bridges Epidermoid sheets Fibrotic stromal respone

The hystologic subtypes of squamous cell carcinoma include papillary, clear cell, small cell, and basaloid variants and four variants are included, which may be the predominat feature of the tumor but more often may be focal. Spindle cell (squamous) carcinoma is lastly classified as pleomorphic carcinoma under carcinomas with pleomorfic, sarcomatoid or sarcomatous elements.

Papillary variant: This arises in large bronchi, grows endo-bronchially, and may branch at the bronchial bifurcation, extending along bronchial lumina with minimally invasive growth. A verrucous growth pattern may be noted (Dulmet-Brender et al., 1986; Sherwin et al., 1962).

Clear cell variant: Clear changes may be seen in squamous cell carcinoma (Churg et al., 1980).

Small cell variant: This is composed of small cells lacking the characteristics nuclear features of small cell carcinoma, and possessing coarsely granular nuclei, some visible nucleoli and cytoplasm, often with distinct cell borders and focally intercellular bridges (Churg et al., 1980).

Basaloid variant: This is characterized by prominent palisanding of cells at the periphery of the tumor cells nests and by the presence of squamous cell differentiation in some parts (Travis et al., 1999).

1.4. The Anatomic Level

Squamous cell carcinomas of the lung are among the most common of the central airways tumors and accounts for approximately 30% of all lung cancer (Parkin et al., 1999). Two-thirds SCC present as central lung tumors, whereas many among the remaining one-third are peripheral (Colby et al., 1995; Tomashefski et al., 1990).

Squamous cell carcinoma arises most often in segmental bronchi and the involvement of lobar and mainstem bronchi occur by extension (Melamed et al., 1977). Typically, squamous carcinomas spread directly through and replace tissue at the interface between normal lung and carcinoma. Squamous carcinomas can frequently be found spreading through the alveolar septae rather than along the surfaces of the alveolar walls.

Invasive squamous tumors are characterized by the extension of squamous cells beyond the basement membrane of the airway lining.

Invasive squamous carcinoma is recognized as angulated nests or individual tumor cells that have broken away from the surface epithelium and become embedded in the stromal tissues. The invasive cells may form keratin pearls and intercellular bridges and may develop irregular areas of central necrosis described as geographic necrosis. Typically, squamous carcinomas spread directly through and replace tissue at the interface between normal lung and carcinoma. Squamous carcinomas can frequently be found spreading through the alveolar septae rather than along the surfaces of the alveolar septae walls as is observed in bronchioloalveolar carcinomas.

1.5. Immunohistochemical Changes

A variety of molecular mechanisms are thought to be involved in the transformation of in situ lesions to invasive carcinoma. These include changes in the patterns of expression of matrix metalloproteases (MMP) and collagens (Galateau-Salle et al., 2000). Collagen IV and MMP2 are reduced as squamous cells acquire invasive properties while MMP9 is increased (Galateau-Salle et al., 2000; Cox et al., 2000).

One diagnostic marker that is useful in a specific clinical context is cytokeratin. Squamous carcinoma consistently express cytokeratin and can be distinguished from non-epithelial malignancies by the application of pancytokeratin antibodies such as an AE1/AE3 cocktail. Cytokeratin subtype CK5/6 (Ordoñez, 1992; Chu & Weiss, 2002) is also expressed frequently, but unlike adenocarcinoma, squamous tumors rarely express CK7 (Lyda & Weiss, 2000; Chu et al., 2000).

Pre-malignant squamous lesions in the lower airways are associated with changes in protein expression, including overexpression of cytokeratin 5/6 (Ordoñez, 1992; Chu & Weiss, 2002).

2. SQUAMOUS CELL CARCINOMA OF THE HEAD AND NECK

Head and neck squamous cell carcinoma (HNSCC) is a heterogeneous disease with complex molecular alterations. It arises from a cancer progenitor or stem cell followed by outgrowth of clonal populations with cumulative alterations and phenotypic progression to invasive malignancy.

Major risk factors include tobacco use and alcohol abuse in developed countries and betel quid chewing and bidi smoking in Asiantic countries. The casual link between human papillomavirus (HPV) and a subset of HNSCC cases has become established in recent years.

2.1. The Genetic Level

Cancer arises in a multi-step process resulting from the sequential accumulation of genetic and epigenetic defects and the clonal expansion of survivor cell populations (Hanahan & Weinberg, 2000). In the case of HNSCC (Table III), tumor progression involves genetic alterations leading to dysplasia (9p21, 3p21, 17p13), carcinoma in situ (11q13, 13q21, 14q31) and invasive tumors (4q26-28, 6p, 8p, 8q) (Califano et al., 1996). In particular, loss of 9p21 or 3p21 is one of the earliest detectable events leading to the progression to dysplasia. From dysplasia, further genetic alteration in 11q, 13q, 1q creates carcinoma in situ (Califano et al., 1996).

These and several studies suggest the contribution of several known tumor suppressor genes in HNSCC, such as p16 and p14^{ARF} (9p21), which are responsible for G1 cell cycle regulation and MDM2 mediated degradation of p53, respectively, APC (5q21-22) and P53 (17p13), as well as the existence of many putative tumor suppressor genes affected in HNSCC, including FHIT (3p14), and RASSF1 (3p21) (Hunter et al., 2005). Among them, loss of chromosomal region 9p21 is found in 70-80% of dysplastic lesions of the oral mucosa, and together with the inactivation of the remaining alleles of p16 and p14^{ARF} by promoter hypermethylation; represent one of the earliest and most frequent events in HNSSC progression (Califano et al., 1996; Forastiere et al., 2001).

Table 3. Genetic abnormalities that occur in the multi-step carcinogenesis from normal epithelium to squamous cell carcinoma

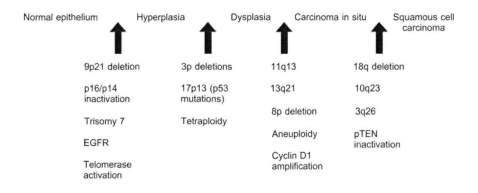

Normal epithelium	Hyperplasia	Dysplasia	Carcinoma in situ	Squamous cell carcinoma
9p21 deletion	3p deletions	11q13	18q deletion	
p16/p14 inactivation	17p13 (p53 mutations)	13q21	10q23	
Trisomy 7	Tetraploidy	8p deletion	3q26	
EGFR		Aneuploidy	pTEN inactivation	
Telomerase activation		Cyclin D1 amplification		

2.2. The Molecular and Cellular Level

Normal cells proliferate only when needed, as a result of a delicate balance between growth- promoting factors and growth- inhibiting signaling under the influence of molecular cues.

An emerging concept is that several activating and inactivating events must occurs in oncogenes and tumor suppressor genes for the initiation and progression of many types of cancer. In HNSCC, these genetic changes occur in a multi-step process (Partridge et al., 1997).

The ability to proliferate continuosly, without undergoing senescene, is one of the hallmarks of cancer (Hanahan & Weinberg, 2000). In HNSCC, limitless replicative potential is most likely acquired trhrough the genetic and epigenetic inactivation of p16, together with mutations in p53 and enhanced activity of the telomerase (Todd et al., 2002). The lack of a functional p16 enables cells to bypass replicative stress-induced senescence (Collado et al., 2007), while the enhanced telomerase activity prevents the shortening of the telomeres and the consequent generation of signals from uncapped telomeres that impinge on p53 and other molecules involved in DNA-damage response (Collado et al., 2007).

Most HNSCCs lose the ability to restrain aberrant growth primarly due to the inactivation of p16, whose normal function is to block cyclin-bound cyclin-dependent kinases (CDKs) CDKa and CDK6 (Weinberg, 1995). The latter orchestrates cell cycle progression and represses the growth inhibitory activity of the retinoblastoma (RB1) gene product (Weinberg, 1995).

RB1 mutations are rare in HNSCC, but a loss of RB in pre-malignant and advanced oral cancer lesions have been reported with variable rates (Pande et al., 1998; Pavelic et al., 1996; Xu et al., 1998) reflecting perhaps that in the presence of p16 inactivation, further mutations or alterations in the p16-Rb tumor suppressor pathway would have a limited growth advantage.

Epidermal growth factor receptor (EGFR) signaling has been strongly implicated in carcinogenesis, and tumor progression in HNSCC. In HNSCC, EGFR is overexpressed in up to 80-100% of tumors (Grandis & Tweardy, 1993), some of the highest rates on any human carcinoma. Interestingly, there are regional differences among tissues in the head and neck that express EGFR, with relatively lower levels associated with laryngeal tumors as compared to those of the oral cavity and oropharynx (Takes et al., 1998).

The predominate mechanims leading to EGFR is overexpression in EGFR gene amplification, with more than 12 copies per cell reported in HNSCC (Teman et al., 2007). Constitutive EGFR activation in HNSCC is also caused by its autocrine stimulation through the co-expression of EGFR with one of its ligands, TGF-α, which is frequently observed in HNSCC (Quon et al., 2001).

EGFR demonstrates increased overexpression in the more advanced-staged carcinomas as well as in those carracinomas that were found to be poorly differentiated (Kaluyankrishna & Grandis, 2006).

Specific mutations of the EGFR receptor have also reported. The most common mutation of EGFR is likely EGFR*VIII*, ocurring in up to 40% of HNSCC (Sok et al., 2006). This mutant receptor is only found in cancer cells and manifests from an in-frame deletion of exons 2-7, which encodes the receptor's extracellular domain, thus resulting in a constitutively active receptor that is completely independent of any activation via ligand binding (Sok et al., 2006).

In addition to overexpression, other pathological manifestations of EGFR can be carried out through mutational activation, amplification, and transactivation by other tyrosine kinases (Karamouzis et al., 2007).

2.3. The Cellular and Histological Level

The mucosal layer consists of a squamous epithelial layer and its basement layer. The squamous layer consists primarily of squamous cells. Associated with healthy squamous cells is an intracellular and extracellular matrix made up of various proteins including keratin, actin, and collagen. The inside of a squamous cell is filled with cytoplasm as well as cell nucleus and other numerous other structures such as mitochondria, Golgi apparatus, endoplasmic reticula, lysosomes, and peroxisomes. There is also a certain amount of keratin-rich material that is generated during the cell's lifetime. This keratin-rich material becomes the dominant material remaining in the cell as the squamous epithelial cell approaches apoptosis.

The submucosal layer consists of numerous cell types. The strength of the layer is due to the long collagen fibers that crisscross the latter parallel to the mucosal surface. Such a crisscossed layer can be referred to as a lamina propia. These collagen fibers are hollow and have an index contrast on the order of the nuclei from the cell.

Pre-malignant and malignant lesions arise most frequently from epithelium, and these epithelial lesions ultimately account for 95% of all cancers of the oral cavity.

Erythroplakia is characteristically defined as a velvety red patch that cannot be clinically or pathologically ascribed to any specific disease entity. Epithelial dysplasia is a pre-malignant condition characterized clinically by an alteration in the oral epithelium that may cause the oral mucosa to turn red, white, or some other color variation. Dysplasia is generally classified, microscopically, as mild, moderate, or severe. The risk of transformation of oral epithelial dysplasia to squamous cell cancer has been reported to be as 25%, a much higher transformation rate than 5% reported for homogenous leukoplakias (Mashberg & Meyers, 1976).

Carcinoma in situ can present in the oral cavity as a red or white lesion, as some other mucosal discoloration, or as a distinct tumor mass.

A range of histologic features can be identified in squamous cell carcinoma of the oral cavity, but all show a commonality. Clinically, squamous cell carcinoma can present as a red lesion, a white lesion, an ulcer or tumor mass, or some other variation or color. The basement membrane (BM) of the oral epithelium is violated in all cases of squamous cell carcinoma, and the neoplastic process extends beyond the BM into the connective tissue lamina propia as broad sheets, nests, cords, and islands of neoplastic cells of epithelial origin.

Histologically, oral squamous cell carcinomas are typically categorized as well- differentiated, moderately- differentiated, poorly- differentiated, or undifferentiated. The well-differentiated neoplasm are generally with minimal cellular atypia and mytotic atypia, round oval nuclei with eosinophilic cytoplasm and intracellular bridging; keratin formation is a common feature associated with well-differentiated squamous cell carcinomas, as is individual cell keratinization and a loss of attachment between cells. The poorly-differentiated neoplasms are rarely seen with ccytokeratin staining. The undifferentiated neoplasms are often referred to as non-keratinizing squamous cell carcinomas.

2.4. The Anatomic Level

The anatomic site of presentation of HNSCC can be of considerable significance in a patient's prognosis. Squamous cell carcinomas of the oral cavity demonstrated that tumors of equal size that involved the lip, buccal mucosa, hard palate, and the gingiva had a similar risk of metastatic spread to regional lymph nodes (Shear et al., 1976).

2.5. Immunohistochemical Changes

Cytokeratins (CKs) are the intermediate filament proteins of the epithelium cells, which have become important markers of normal and abnormal cell differentiation. CKs alterations have been reported in carcinomas from different anatomical sites, and these have been associated with specific aspects of tumor behavior (Depont et al., 1999) and related to the cellular differentiation level. The normal pattern shows the keratin pair K5/14 in the stratum basal whereas K1/10, or K4/13, are the two pairs associated with differentiating suprabasal cells (Heyden et al., 1992).

In HNSCC, immunoreactivity for cytokeratins were reported as variable pattern. Tumors with reduced α-catenin expression showed a uniformly negative pattern more frequently thant a heterogeneous pattern. It has been reported that cadherins associated with at least three distinct cytoplasmic proteins, termed catenins (Ozawa et al., 1990). Catenins have been classified into α, β and γ-catenin. The adhesive function of cadherins is dependent on their association with cytoplasmic regulatory proteins, the best characterized of which are α-catenin, β-catenin and γ-catenin (also known as plakoglobin)

(Hülsken et al., 1994). In HNSCC, reduced catenin staining was found in all tumors, but there was no evidence for coordinated regulation of expression of α-, β- and γ-catenin (Andrews et al., 1997; Bagutti et al., 1998).

3. THE WNT AND B-CATENIN LIAISE

The β-catenin gene maps to 3p21 and encodes a 92- to 97-kd protein, that it participates in two disparate cellular functios: the first concerns homotypic cell-cell interactions, by complexing with E-cadherin, whereas, the second one involves signal transduction pathways that are activated by the Wnt, the integrin-associated tyrosine kinases, integrin-linked kinase, and focal adhesion kinase, as well as presenilins.

Cytoplasmic β-catenin that is not incorporatdes in cell adhesion or signaling, is regulated by two proteasome degradation complexes. The first complex, suspected to be the deault mechanisms, requires GSK-3β-dependent phosporylation of β-catenin at N-terminus for destruction. The second complex, responds to p53-induced cell cycle arrest. Both mechanisms require APC as a scaffold. APC binds β-catenin in the central third and not only mediates its degradation, but also regulates its subcellular localization.

An increase in β-catenin cytoplasmic levels, after stimulation from Wnt signaling pathway, results in its nuclear accumulation. There, it heterodimerizes with members of the lymphoid enhancer factor/T-cell factor family of transcription factors and activates the expression of a broad pattern of target genes.

High levels of β-catenin that result from mutations in genes coding for components of the degradation systems, mutations in β-catenin, or deregulated Wnt signaling, are stabilized in the cytoplasm, leading to an increased β-catenin nuclear accumulation. As a consequence, β-catenin exerts oncogenic activity through aberrant target gene expression.

Among the many molecular markers associated with tumor progression, the Wnt family has been shown to encode the multi-functional signaling glycoproteins that are involved in the regulation of a wide variety of normal and pathologic processes, including embriogenesis, differentiation, and tumorigenesis.

3.1. Wnt Expression in NSCLC and HNSCC

In the human adult lung, Wnt2, Wnt5A, and Wnt11 are expressed in the mesenchyme and Wnt7 is expressed in lung epithelium (Wang et al., 2005; Lako et al., 1998; Shu et al., 2002; Li et al., 2002). The Wnt pathway plays a critical role in lung carcinogenesis, and aberrant Wnt pathway has been shown to have a role in non-small cell lung cancer (NSCLC) (Uematsu et al., 2003) (Figure 1 and 2). In fact, many previous clinical studies have demonstrated that Wnt5a expression is frequently up regulated in various human cancers.

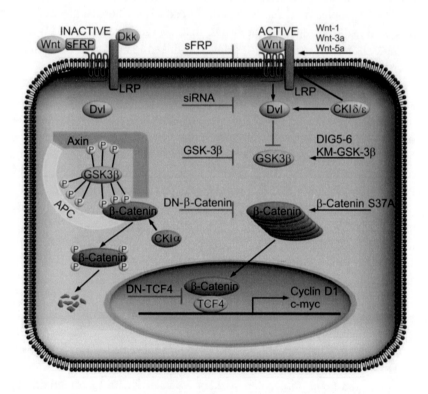

Figure 1. Active and inactive Wnt/Wingless signaling pathway. In the inactive Wnt pathway, β-catenin forms a complex with Axin and APC and, after phosphorylation by CK1a and GSK-3, β-catenin is degraded by ubiquitination. Active Wnt pathway there leads to inhibition of β-catenin degradation and its accumulation in the cytoplasm.

As a result, the overexpression of Wnt5a might affect tumor biology during tumor progression. The temporal and spatial patterns of Wnt-5A expression are quite complex during embryonic development: in contrast, in the adult, expression is restricted to the lungs, heart and brain (Li et al., 2002). Wnt-5A gene is mapped to chrosomosome 3p14-p21 (Clark et al., 1993).

Many years ago, search on a panel of human tumors (Lozzo et al., 1995), discovered the role for Wnt-5A expression in lung carcinoma, and their findings indicate that the Wnt-5A gene are operational both during development and neoplastic growth, suggesting that Wnt-5A protein may contribute to the maintenance of the transformed phenotype *in vivo*.

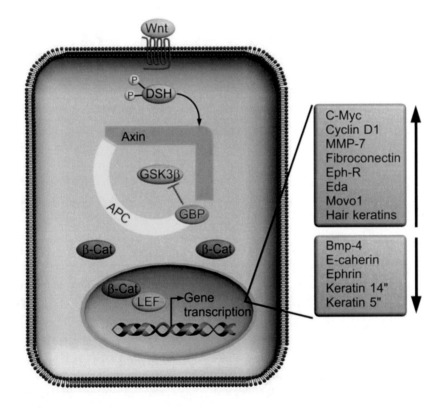

Figure 2. Wnt signaling pathway promotes the transcription of genes involved in cell proliferation or apoptosis inhibition.

Later, it was shown that Wnt5a gene expression in squamous cell carcinoma of the lung was significantly higher than that in adenocarcinoma, and demonstrated that Wnt5a status isto be a significant factor (Huang et al., 2005). Regarding the expression patterns of intratumoral β-catenin related to stromal β-catenin expression, the percentage of β-catenin positive stromal cells was significantly higher in Wnt5a-positive tumors than in Wnt5a-negative tumors (Huang et al., 2005).

AlthoughWhereas activation of Wnt-β-catenin pathway is a frequent event in many different human tumors, there is limited knowledge on the contribution of this signaling mechanims in HNSCC. However, we now know that several comnponents of the Wnt pathway are also altered in oral cancers. Several Wnt receptors, Frizzleds, and their downstream target, Dishevelled, are highly expressed in HNSCC when compared to matching normal (Leethanakul et al., 2009), and high levels of Wnt14 were detected in microdissected HNSCC cells. On the other hand, reduced expression of natural Wnt antagonists is a frequent epigenetic event in HNSCC (Marsit et al., 2006).

Deregulated action of the APC tumor suppressor protein is often compromised in HNSCC by the loss of heterozygosity (LOH) and hypermethylation of the APC gene and its consequent reduced expression level (Worsham et al., 2006; Chang et al., 2000).

The normal epithelium showed only a few positive cells in the basal/parabasal layers. Positive staining was always granular, which localized in the cytoplasm, and had a striking membrane outline. The staining of Wnt1 in hyperplastic and dysplastic oral epithelium was mainly located in the parabasal layers diffusing into the cytopasm (Lo Muzio et al., 2002).

Most of the well-differentiated HNSCC showed cell positivity for Wnt1. Positive cells were preferentially localized in the parabasal layers, often in the central areas, and rarely in the basal layer stained with Wnt1. In most cases of moderatly- and poorly-differentieted HNSCC, few cells are found positive, including the invading front of the tumors (Lo Muzio et al., 2002). The expression of Wnt1 is correlated with those of β-catenin and γ-catenin in HNSCC.

These findings suggest the existence of a subgroup of HNSCC in which the Wnt pathway may be related to oral carcinogenesis. The expression of β-catenin is altered in HNSCC (Ueda et al., 2006; Mahomed et al., 2007), even though no activating mutations in this molecule have yet identified (Lo Muzio et al., 2005).

3.2. B-Catenin

β-catenin is a protein which interacts with the cytoplasmic domain of E-cadherin and with α-catenin, anchoring the cadherin complex to the actin cytoskeleton (Kemler & Ozawa, 1999) (Figure 3 and 4). β-catenin activity is controlled by a large number of binding partners that affect the stability and localization of β-catenin. The stability of β-catenin, encoded by the gene CTNNB1, is regulated by a multi-protein complex consisting of β-catenin, Axin/Conductin, APC, and GSK-3β (Schwarz-Romond et al., 2002). In the Wnt signaling pathway, β-catenin plays a key role as a transcriptional activation conjunction with lymphoid-enhancer factor /T cell DNA-binding protein to induce target gene expression resulting in cell proliferation and differentiation.

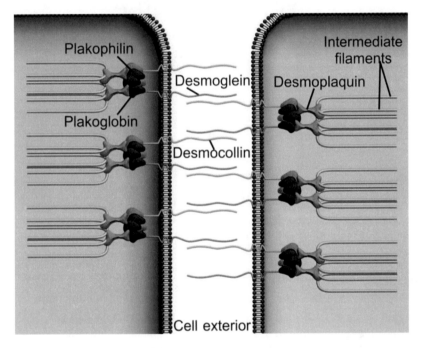

Figure 3. Desmosomal-type junction and its components: α-, β- and γ-catenin.

The primary structure of β-catenin is compriseds of an amino-terminal domain of approximately 130 amino acids, a central region of 12 imperfect reppeats of 42 amino acids known as arm repeats, and carboxy-terminal domain of 110 amino acids. The amino-terminus of β-catenin is important for regulating of its stability, whereas the carboxyl terminus works as a transcriptional activator domain (Willert & Nusse, 1998).

γ-catenin, also called plakoglobin, shares overall 70% amino acid identity with β-catenin and as much as 80% within the arm repeat domain (Huber & Weis, 2001). Plakoglobin binds E-cadherin, α-catenin, APC, Axib and Tcf/Lef transcription factors, and is involved in cell adhesion as well as Wnt signaling. However, differences between β-catenin and plakoglobin in these processes exist (Kolligs et al., 2000).

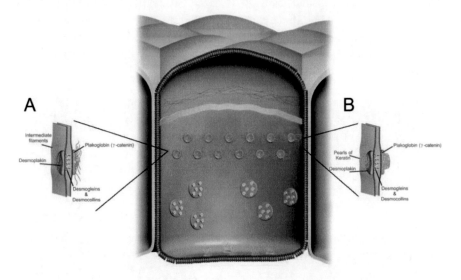

Figure 4. Epithelium showing the different types of intercellular junctions. A, normal structure of the desmosome. B, pathological structure of the desmosome where an accumulation of β-catenin in the form of keratin pearls could be observed.

α-catenin, a protein involved in cell adhesion by anchoring the β-catenin/E-cadherin complex to the actin cytoskeleton, are encoded in the CTNNA1 gene. Binding of α-catenin to the N-terminal region of β-catenin (Nagafuchi et al., 1994) and E-cadherin to the arm repeat (Huber & Weis, 2001) connects β-catenin to cell adhesion.

E-cadherin, encoding by the CDH1 gene, is a calcium-dependent transmembrane glycoprotein, localizsed to zonula adherens junctions at the basolateral surface in epithelial cells and is involved in cell-cell interaction. Normal E-cadherin expression plays a key role in the maintenance of epithelial integrity and polarity function. The E-cadherin molecule is composed of a cytoplasmic domain, a single-pass transmembrane domain and an extracellular domain that consists of five tandemly repeat cadherin-motifs subdomains with putative calcium-binding sites. The cytoplasmic domain of E-cadherin interacts with the catenin molecules that mediate its binding to the actin cytoskeleton.

3.2.1. A-Catenin, B-Catenin, And Γ-Catenin Expression in Normal Skin/ Epithelium

The intensity of staining for β-catenins increased from the basal/parabasal layers towards the intermediate malpighian layer. No staining was observed in the upper layer.

The pattern of staining was prevalently membranous, with a progressive displacement of the signal towards the periphery of the cells from basal to superficial layers. A diffused, cytoplasmic staining was observed focally in the parabasal layers. This variation of the staining pattern presumablye could be due to the progressive intracellular accumulation of keratins from the less-differentiated basal layers towards the fully-keratinized superficial layers. No staining was observed in stromal structures. Normal skin was characterized by an intense membranous staining for β-catenin, with a progressive displacement of the signal toward the periphery of the cells.

The β-catenin expression is membranous in normal epithelium. Positive staining of the two proteins is mainly observed in the parabasal layers of epithelium.

3.2.2. B-Catenin in NSCLC and HNSCC

β-catenin is a versatile component of homotypic cell adhesion and signaling. Its subcellular localization and cytoplasmic levels are tightly regulated by the adenomatous polyposis coli (APC) protein. In tumor cells, β-catenin generally exhibited homogeneous staining with four expression patterns (Kotsinas et al., 2002).

Mutations in β-catenin or APC result in β-catenin aberrant over-expression that is associated with its nuclear accumulation and improper gene activation (Figure 5 and 6).

Data from experimental models have shown that β-catenin overexpression has a multitude of effects on cell-cycle behavior. In many of these aspects, its function depends on major G1 phase regulators.

However, given their dual cellular function, different expression patterns have been reported not only among distinct types of cancer, but also between tumors of the same origin (Grabsh et al., 2001; Billim et al., 2000; Papadavid et al., 2001; Brabletz et al., 2000).

Membranous localization of β-catenin is frequently interpreted as an association with E-cadherin-dependent cell adhesion. In such cases, a loss or reduction in staining correlates with tumor dedifferentiation, infiltrative growth, metastases, and poor prognosis (Christofori & Semb, 1999). On the other, nuclear and/or cytoplasmic presence has been correlated with β-catenin or APC mutations (Polakis, 2000). Aberrant expression of β-catenin has been reported in a variety of cancers (Polakis, 2000).

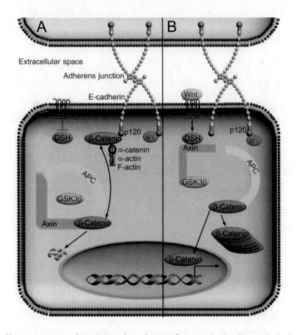

Figure 5. In cells not exposed to Wnt signal (A), β-catenin is degraded through the ubiquitin pathway after phosphorylation by GSK-3. On the contrary, in cells exposed to Wnt signal (B), the interaction between Dsh and Axin provokes the inhibition of GSK that prevents β-catenin phosphorylation; resulting in its accumulation and its entrance into the nucleus to increase the transcription activity.

For well-differentiated HNSCC, the intensity of staining for β-catenin, and γ-catenin increased from peripheral layers toward the central part of the cancer nests. A diffuse cytoplasmic staining for β-catenin and γ-catenin are observed focally. For moderately- and poorly-differentiated HNSCC, cancer cells in a few cases are found positive for β-catenin and γ-catenin, including the invading front of the tumors.

Investigation β-catenin expression in NSCLC demonstrated a subset of non-small-cell lung carcinomas that showed different patterns of β-catenin performance (Kotsinas et al., 2002). Four β-catenin immunohistochemical expression patterns: membranous 11.1%, membranous-cytoplasmic 54.3%, cytoplasmic 9.9%, cytoplasmic-nuclear 24.7% were observed. The presence of β-catenin in the cytoplasm is an indication of aberrant expression; the cases with nuclear β-catenin expression represents a subset of NSCLC that have gained an increased proliferation advantage (Kotsinas et al., 2002).

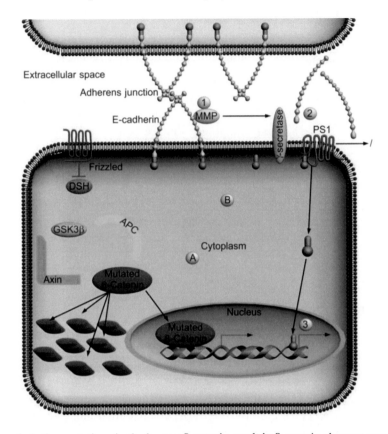

Figure 6. Active mutations in the human β-catenin result in β-catenin aberrant over-expression that is associated with its nuclear accumulation and improper gene activation .

Expression of all three catenins (α, β, γ) is related to histological type and differentiation in NSCLC, although catenins have no independent value (Pirinen et al., 2001). Normal catenin staining was found significantly more often in adenocarcinomas than in squamous cell carcinomas or anaplastic/large cell carcinomas. The tumors with reduced staining of β-catenin and γ-catenin were found in 7% and 23% cases, respectively (Pirinen et al., 2001). In NSCLC, reduced expression of β-catenins and γ-catenin has been related to poor prognosis (Pantel et al., 1998; Retera et al., 1998).

Reduced β-catenin expression in surgically treated NSCLC is clearly associated with lymph node metastasis and an unfavorable prognosis: the expression of β-catenin in primary NSCLC is inversely correlated with the presence of lymph node metastases (Retera et al., 1998).

In addition, supraglottic tumors showed more often cytoplasmic involvement α-catenin than glottic tumors (Hirvikoski et al., 1998). Reduced expression of γ-catenin is associated with dedifferentiation in primary SCC of the oropharynx and hypopharynx (Pukkila et al., 2001). The expression of K8/18 in SCCs of the oral cavity is an independent prognostic marker and indicates a decreased overall and progression free survival (PFS) (Fillies et al., 2006).

Correlation of E-cadherin and β-catenin expression in NSCLC demonstrated clinical significance: reduced E-cadherin expression was noted in 42% and reduced β-catenin expression was evident in 37% of cases (Kase et al., 2000). These results are correlated with poor prognosis. Multi-variate analysis showed a significant lower survival rate for patients with reduced β-catenin (Kase et al., 2000).

3.3. Wnt Signaling and B-Catenin Stabilization

The Wnt5a protein can act via Frz-5 receptor to initiate an intracellular pathway leading to the accumulation of β-catenin.

Wnt porteins are closely associated with the cell surface (Papkoff & Schryver, 1990) and the extracellular matrix (Bradley & Brown, 1990), where they interact with heparan sulfate in the pericellular environment (Kiefer et al., 1991).

The Wnt proteins also share the ability to induce cell proliferation via an autocrine or paracrine route, which appears to be mediated by a direct effect of Wnt proteins on stabilizing adhesion molecules such as plakoglobin and E-cadherin (Bradley et al., 1993). This suggested the existence of a tumor-stromal interaction. In benign tumors, stromal proliferation is under the control of the epithelium. Although the epithelium promotes stromal growth, it also limits it in benign tumors, because any excesive stromal growth alters the epithelium: stroma ratio.

The Wnt signal stabilizes β-catenin protein and determines its accumulation in the cytoplasma and nucleus.

While normal skin cells showed a Wnt1 positive staining only of the cutaneous annexa and few cells in the basal/parabasal layers, in basal cell carcinomas (BCCs), the areas of de-differentiation showed a high granular positive staining (>50% of cells).

3.4. Expression of Cytokeratins 5/14 in SCC

Under normal circumnstances, the gene KRT5 and KRT14 genes code for keratin 5 and keratin 14, rescpectively. The KRT5 gene is located on chromosome 12q12-q13 and don´t forget chromosome 17q12-q21, home of KRT14. Keratins 5 and 14 naturally partner together. A second natural partner for keratin 5 is keratin 15 that is more abundantly expressed in internal stratified squamous epithelium.

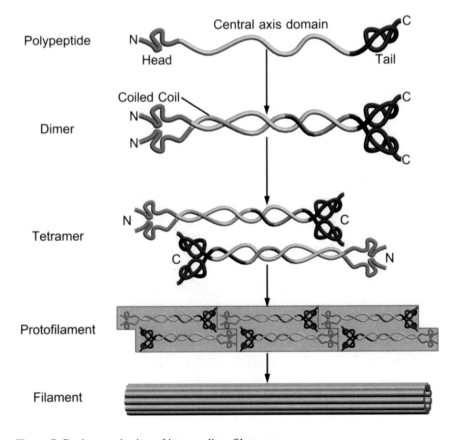

Figure 7. Basic constitution of intermediate filaments.

Withinhitin the cell are three types of cytoskeletal elements: microtubules, thin filaments (actin), and intermediate filaments. These elements work together to provide stability to the cell. Of the five different types of intermediate filaments, keratins comprise two. These include the basic and acidic keratins. Many keratins form copolymners and they dimerize in coiled-coil interactions (Figure 7).

Cytokeratin 5/14 are expressed in the basal layer of stratified epithelia. The keratin networks formed by keratins 5 and 14 can be comprised of up to 25% of the cell´s content (Chu et al., 2001).

Cytokeratin 5/6 are intermediate-sized basic keratins. In normal tissue, cytokeratin 5/6 are mainly expressed in keratinizing (epidermis) and non-keratinizing (mucosa) squamous epithelium. Cytokeratin 5/6 immunoreactivity has been observed in the majority of cases of squamous cell carcinoma (Chu et al., 2002).

CONCLUSIONS

Intermediate filaments are central components of the intracellular skeleton. The expression of distinct intermediate filament proteins is tissue-specific and almost highly conserved during carcinogenesis. Several studies associated changes in intermediate filament expression with an altered cellular behavior.

The expression of high molecular weight cytokeratins, especially CK5, is a hallmark of squamous epithelium and is predominantly seen in the basal layer of stratified epithelium. This cell layer is regarded as the anatomical localization of tissue specific stem/progenitor cells. Stem cells of stratified epithelium have been repeatedly described as the major cellular targets for cancer causing mutations and therefore might give in a long term rise to the development of SCCs of lung and/or head and neck organs.

ACKNOWLEDGMENT

Silvia Díaz Prado is supported by an Isidro Parga Pondal contract from Xunta de Galicia, A Coruña (Spain).

REFERENCES

Andrews NA, Jones AS, Helliwell TR, Kinsella AR. Expression of the E-cadherin-catenin cell adhesion complex in primary squamous cell carcinomas of the head and neck and their nodal metastases. *Br J Cancer* 1997; 75:1474-80.

Auerbach O, Stout AP, Hammond EC, Garfinkel L. Changes in bronchial epithelium in relation to sex, age, residence, smoking and pneumonia. *N Engl J Med* 1962; 267:111-9.

Bagutti C, Speight PM, Watt FM. Comparison of integrin, cadherin, and catenin expression in squamous cell carcinomas of the oral cavity. *J Pathol* 1998; 186:8-16.

Balsara BR, Sonoda G, du Manoir S, Siegfried JM, Gabrielson E, Testa JR. Comparative genomic hybridization analysis detects frequent, often high-level, over-representation of DNA sequences at 3q, 5p, 7p, and 8q in human non-small cell lung carcinomas. *Cancer Res* 1997; 57:2116-20.

Balsara BR, Testa JR. Chromosomal imbalances in human lung cancer. *Oncogene* 2002; 21:6877-83.

Billim V, Kawasaki T, Katagari A, Wakatsuki S, Takahashi K, Tomita Y. Altered expression of β-catenin in renal cell cancer and transitional cell cancer with the absence of β-catenin gene mutations. *Clin Cancer Res* 2000; 6:460-6.

Brabletz T, Hermann K, Jung A, Faller G, Kirchner T. Expression of nuclear beta-catenin and c-myc is correlated with tumor size but not with proliferative activity of colorectal adenomas. *Am J Pathol* 2000; 156:865-70.

Bradley RS, Brown AMC. The proto-oncogene int-1 encodes a secreted protein associated with the extracellular matrix. *EMBO J* 1990; 9:2569-75.

Bradley RS, Cowin P, Brown AMC. Expression of Wnt-1 in PC12 cells results in modulation of plakoglobin and E-cadherin and increased cellular adhesion. *J Cell Biol* 1993; 123:1857-65.

Califano J, van der Riet P, Westra W, Nawroz H, Clayman G, Piantadosi S, Corio R, Lee D, Greenberg B, Koch W, Sidransky D. Genetic progression model for head and neck cancer: implications for field cancerization. *Cancer Res* 1996; 56:2488-92.

Carlile A, Edwards C. Poorly differentiated squamous carcinoma of the bronchus: a light and electron microscopic study. *J Clin pathol* 1986; 39:284-92.

Carter D. Squamous cell carcinoma of the lung: an update. *Semin Diagn Pathol* 1985; 2:226-34.

Chang KW, Lin SC, Mangold KA, Jean MS, Yuan TC, Lin SN, Chang CS. Alterations of adenomatous polyposis coli (APC) gene in oral squamous cell carcinoma. *Int J Oral Maxillofac Surg* 2000; 29:223-6.

Chaudhuri MR. Primary pulmonary cavitating carcinomas. *Thorax* 1973; 28:354-66.

Christofori G, Semb H. The role of the cell-adhesion molecule E-cadherin as a tumor-suppressor gene. *Trends Biochem Sci* 1999; 24:73-6.

Chu P, Wu E, Weiss LM. Cytokeratin 7 and cytokeratin 20 expression in epithelial neoplasms: a survey of 435 cases. *Mod Pathol* 2000; 13:962-72.

Chu PG, Lyda MH, Weiss LM. Cytokeratin 14 expression in epithelial neoplasms: a survey of 435 cases with emphasis on its value in differentiating squamous cell carcinomas from other epithelial neoplasms. *Histopathology* 2001; 39:9-16.

Chu PG, Weiss LM. Expression of cytokeratin5/6 in epithelial neoplasms: an immunohistochemical study of 509 cases. *Mod Pathol* 2002; 15:6-10.

Churg A, Johnston WH, Stulbarg M. Small cell squamous and mixed small cell squamous-small cell anaplastic carcinomas of the lung. *Am J Surg Pathol* 1980; 4:255-63.

Clark CC, Cohen I, Eichstetter I, Cannizaro LA, McPherson JD, Wasmuth JJ, Iozzo RV. Molecular cloining of the human proto-oncogene Wnt-5A and mapping of the gene (WNT5A) to chromosome 3p14-p21. *Genomics* 1993; 18:249-60.

Colby TV, Koss MN, Travis WD. *Tumors of the lower respiratory tract; Armed Forces Institute of Pathology fascicle*. Third Series. Washington, DC, :Armed Forces Institute of Patholoy, 1995.

Collado M, Blasco MA, Serrano M. Cellular senesence in cancer and aging. *Cell* 2007; 130:223-33.

Cox G, Jones JL, O´Byerne KF. Matrix metalloproteinase 9 and the pidermal growth factor signal pathways in operable non-small cell lung cancer. *Clin Cancer Res* 2000; 6:2349-55.

Depont J, Shabana AH, Sawaf H, Gehanno P, Forest N. Cytokeratin alterations as diagnostic and prognostic markers of oral and pharyngeal carcinomas. A prospective study. *Eur J Oral Sci* 1999; 107:442-54.

Dulmet-Brender E, Jaubert F, Huchon G. Exophytic endobronchial epidermoid carcinoma. *Cancer* 1986; 57:1358-64.

Fillies T, Werkmeister R, Packeisen J, Brandt B, Morin P, Weingart D, Joos U, Buerger H. Cytokeratin 8/18 expression indicates a poor prognosis in squamous cell carcinomas of the oral cavity. *BMC Cancer* 2006; 6:10-7.

Forastiere A, Koch W, Trotti A, Sidransku D. Head and neck cancer. *N Engl J Med* 2001; 345:1890-900.

Galateau-Salle FB, Luna RE, Horiba K, Sheppard MN, Hayashi T, Fleming MV, Colby TV, Bennett W, Harris CC, Stetler-Stevenson WG, Liotta L, Ferrans VJ, Travis WD. Matrix metalloproteinases and tissue inhibitors of metalloproteinases in bronchial squamous preinvasive. *Hum Pathol* 2000; 31:296-305.

Girard L, Zöchbauer-Müller S, Virmani AK, Gazdar AF, Minna JD. Genome-wide allelotyping of lung cancer identifies new regions of allelic loss, differences between small cell lung cancer and non-small cell lung cancer, and loci clustering. *Cancer Res* 2000; 60:4894-906.

Grabsh H, Takeno S, Noguchi T, Hommel G, Gabbert HE, Mueller W. Different patterns of beta-catenin expression in gastric carcinomas: relationship with clinicopathological parameters and prognostic outcome. *Histopathology* 2001; 39:141-9.

Grandis JR, Tweardy DJ. Elevated levels of transforming growth factor alpha and epidermal growth factor receptor messenger RNA are early markers of carcinogenesis in head and neck cancer. *Cancer Res* 1993; 53:3579-84.

Hanahan D, Weinberg RA. The hallmarks of cancer. Cell 2000; 100:57-70.

Hecht SS. Cigarette smoking and lung cancer: chemical mechanisms and approaches to prevention. *Lancet Oncol* 2002; 3:461-9.

Heyden A, Huitfeldt HS, Koppang HS, Thrane PS, Bryne M, Brandtzaeg P. Cytokeratins as epithelial differentiation markers in pre-malignant and malignant oral lesions. *J Oral Pathol Med* 1992; 21:7-11.

Hirvikoski P, Kumpulainen EJ, Virtaniemi JA, Helin HL, Rantala I, Johansson RT, Juhola M, Kosma V-M. Cytoplasmic accumulation of α-catenin is associated with aggressive features in laryngeal squamous-cell carcinoma. *In J Cancer* 1998; 79:546-50.

Huang C, Liu D, Nakano J, Ishikawa S, Kontani K, Yokomise H, Ueno M. Wnt5a expression is associated with the tumor proliferation and the stromal vascular endothelial growth factor--an expression in non-small-cell lung cancer. *J Clin Oncol* 2005; 23:8765-73.

Huber AH, Weis WI. The structure of the beta-catenin/E-cadherin complex and the molecular basis diverse ligand recognition by beta-catenin. *Cell* 2001; 105:391-402.

Hülsken J, Behrens J, Birchmeier W. Tumor-suppressor gene products in cell contacts: the cadherin-APC-armadillo connection. *Curr Opin Cell Biol* 1994; 6:711-6.

Hunter KD, Parkinson EK, Harrison PR. Profiling early head and neck cancer. *Nat Rev Cancer* 2005; 5:127-35.

Kaluyankrishna S, Grandis JR. Epidermal growth factor receptor biology in head and neck cancer. *J Clin Oncol* 2006; 24:2666-72.

Karamouzis MV, Grandis JR, Argiris A. Therapies directed against epidermal growth factor receptor in aerodigestive carcinomas. *JAMA* 2007; 298:70-82.

Kase S, Sugio K, Yamazaki K, Okamoto T, Yano T, Sugimachi K. Expression of E-cadherin and β-catenin in human non-small cell lung cancer and the clinical significance. *Clin Cancer Res* 2000; 6:4789-96.

Kemler R, Ozawa M. Uvomorulin-catenin complex: cytoplasmic anchorage of a Ca2+-dependent cell adhesion molecule. *BioEssays: new and reviews in molecular, cellular and development biology.* 1999; 11:88-91.

Kiefer P, Peters G, Dickson C. The Int-2/Fgf-3 oncogene product is secreted and associates with extracellular matrix: implications for cell transformation. *Mol Cell Biol* 1991; 11:5929-36.

Kolligs FT, Kolligs B, Hajra KM, Hu G, Tani M, Cho KR, Fearon ER. Gamma-catenin is regulated by the APC-tumor suppressor and its oncogenic activity is distinct from that of beta-catenin. *Genes & Development* 2000; 14:1319-31.

Kotsinas A, Evangelou K, Zacharatos P, Kittas Ch, Gorgoulis VG. Proliferation, but not apoptosis, is associated with distinct β-catenin expression patterns in non-small-cell lung carcinomas. *Am J Pathol* 2002; 161:1619-34.

Lako M, Strachan T, Bullen P, Wilson DI, Robson SC, Lindsay S. Isolation, characterizsation and embryonic expression of Wnt11, a gene which maps to 11q13.5 and has possible roles in the development of skeleton, kidney and lung. *Gene* 1998; 219:101-10.

Leethanakul C, Patel V, Gillespie J, Pallente M, Ensley JF, Koontongkaew S, Liotta LA, Emmert-Buck M. Distinct pattern of expression of differentiation and growth-related genes in squamous cell carcinomas of the head and neck revealed by the use of laser capture microdissection and cDNA arrays. *Oncogene* 2009; 19:3220-4.

Li C, Xiao J, Hormi K, Borok Z, Minoo P. Wnt5a participates in distal lung morphogenesis. *Devlop Biol* 2002; 248:68-81.

Lo Muzio L, Goteri G, Capretti R, Rubini C, Vinella A, Fumarulo R, Bianchi F, Mastrangelo F, Porfiri E, Mariggiò MA. Beta-catenin gene analysis in oral squamous cell carcinoma. *Int J Immunopathol Pharmacol* 2005; 18:33-8.

Lo Muzio L, Pannone G, Staibano S, Mignogna MD, Griego M, Ramires P, Romitos AM, De Rosa G, Piattellui A. Wnt-1 expression in basal cell carcinoma of head and neck. An immunohistochemical and confocal study with regard to the intracellular distribution of beta-catenin. Anticancer Res 2002; 22:565-76.

Lozzo RV, Eichstetter I, Danielson KG. Aberrant expression of the growth factor Wnt-5A in human malignancy. *Cancer Res* 1995; 55:3495-9.

Lyda MH, Weiss LM. Immunoreactivity for epithelial and neuroendocrine antibodies are useful in the differential diagnosis of lung carcinomas. *Hum Pathol* 2000; 31:980-7.

Mahomed F, Altini M, Meer S. Altered E-cadherin/beta-catenin expression in oral squamous carcinoma with and without nodal metastasis. *Oral Dis* 2007; 13:386-92.

Marsit CJ, McClean MD, Furniss CS, Kelsey KT. Epigenetic activation of the SFRP genes is associated with drinking, smoking and HPV in head and neck squamous cell carcinoma. *Int J cancer* 2006; 119:1761-6.

Mashberg A, Meyers H. Anatomical site and size of 222 early asymptomatic oral squamous cell carcinomas: a continuing prospective study of oral cancer. II. *Cancer* 1976; 37:2149.

Massion PP, Kuo WL, Stokoe D, Olshen AB, Treseler PA, Chin K, Chen C, Polikoff D, Jain AN, Pinkel D, Albertson DG, Jablons DM, Gray JW. Genomic copy number analysis of non-small cell lung cancer using array genomic hybridization: implications of the phosphatidylinositol 3-kinase pathway. *Cancer Res* 2002; 62:3636-40.

Melamed MR, Zaman MB, Flehinger BJ,Martini N. Radiologically occult in situ and incipient invasive epidermoid lung cancer: detection by sputum cytology in a survey asymptomatic cigarette smokers. *Am J Surg Pathol* 1977; 1:5-16.

Nagafuchi A, Ishihara S, Tsukita S. The roles of catenins in the cadherin-mediated cell adhesion: functional analysis of E-cadherin-alpha catenin fusion molecules. *J Cell Biol* 1994; 127:235-45.

Ordoñez NG. Value of cytokeratin 5/6 immunostaining in distinguishing epithelial mesothelioma of the pleura from lung adenocarcinoma. *Am J Surg Pathol* 1992; 22:1215-21.

Ozawa M, Ringwald M, Kemler R. Uvomorulin-catenin complex formation is regulated by a specific domain in the cytoplasmic region of the cell adhesion molecule. *Proc Natl Acad Sci USA* 1990; 87:4246-50.

Pande P, Mathur M, Shukla NK, Ralhan R. pRb and p16 protein alterations in human oral tumorigenesis. *Oral Oncol* 1998; 34:396-403.

Pantel K, Passlick B, Vogt J, Stosiek P, Angstwurm M, Seen-Hibler R, Häussinger K, Thetter O, Izbicki JR, Riethmüller G. Reduced expression of plakoglobin indicates unfavorable prognosis in subset of patients with non-small cell lung cancer. *J Clin Oncol* 1998; 16:1407-13.

Papadavid E, Pignatelli M, Zakynthinos S, Krausz T, Chu AC. The potential role of abnormal E-cadherin and alpha-, beta- and gamma-catenin immunoreactivity in the determination of the biological behaviour of keatoacanthoma. *Br J Dermatol* 2001; 145:582-9.

Papkoff J, Schryver B. Secreted int-1 protein is associated with the cell surface. *Mol Cell Biol* 1990; 10:2723-30.

Parkin DM, Pisani P, Ferlay J. Global cancer statistics. CA *Cancer J Clin* 1999; 49:33-64.

Partridge M, Emilion G, Pateromichelakis S, Philips E, Langdon J. Field cancerizsation of the oral cavity: comparison of the spectrum of molecular alterations in cases presenting with both dysplastic and malignant lesions. *Oral Oncol* 1997; 33:332-7.

Pavelic ZP, Lasmar M, Pavelic L, Sorensen C, Stambrook PJ, Zimmerman N, Gluckman JL. Absence of retinoblastoma gene product in human primary oral cavity carcinomas. *Eur J Cancer B Oral Oncol* 1996; 32B:347-51.

Pfeifer GP, Denissenko MF, Olivier M, Tretyakova N, Hecht SS, Hainaut P. Tobacco smoke carcinogens, DNA damage and p53 mutations in smoking-associated cancers. *Oncogene* 2002; 21:7435-51.

Pirinen RT, Hirvikoski P, Johansson RT, Hollmen S, Kosma V-M. Reduced expression of α-catenin, β-catenin, and γ-catenin is associated with high cell proliferative activity and poor differentiation in non-smal cell lung cancer. *J Clin Pathol* 2001; 54:391-5.

Polakis P. Wnt signaling and cancer. *Genes Dev* 2000; 14:1837-51.

Pukkila MJ, Virtaniemi JA, Kumpulainem EJ, Pririnen RT, Johansson RT, Valtonen HJ, Juhola MT, Kosma V-M. Nuclear β-catenin expression is related to unfavourable outcome in oropharyngeal and hypopharyngeal squamous cell carcinoma. *J Clin pathol* 2001;54:42-7.

Quon H, Liu FF, Cummings BJ. Potential molecular prognostic markers in head and neck squamous cell carcinomas. *Head and Neck* 2001; 23:147-59.

Retera JM, Leers MP, Sulzer MA, Theunissen PH. The expression of beta-catenin in non-small-cell lung cancer: a clinicopathological study. *J Clin Pathol* 1998; 51:891-4.

Schwarz-Romond T, Asbrand C, Bakkers J, Kühl M, Schaeffer HJ, Huelsken J, Behrens J, Hammerschmidt M, Birchmeier W. The ankryn repeat protein Diversin recruits Casein kinase Iepsilon to the beta-catenin degradation complex and acts in both canonical Wnt and Wnt/JNK signaling. *Genes & Development* 2002; 16:2073-84.

Shear M, Hawkins DM, Farr HW. The prediction of lymph node metastasis from oral squamous cell carcinoma. *Cancer* 1976;37:1901-7.

Sherwin RP, Laforet EG, Strieder JW. Exophytic endobronchial carcinoma. *J Thorac Cardiovasc Surg* 1962; 43:716-30.

Shu W, Jiang YQ, Lu MM, Morrisey EE. Wnt7b regulates mesenchymal proliferation and vascular development in the lung. *Development* 2002; 129:4831-42.

Sok JC, Coppelli FM, Thomas SM, Lango MN, Xi S, Hunt JL, Freilino ML, Graner MW, Wikstrand CJ, Bigner DD, Gooding WE, Furnari FB, Grandis JR. Mutant epidermal growth factor receptor (EGFRvIII) contributes to head and neck cancer growth and resistance to EGFR targeting. *Clin Cancer Res* 2006; 12:5064-73.

Takes RP, Baatenburg de Jong RJ, Schuurinh E, Litvinov SV, Hermans J, Van Krieken JH. Differences in expression of oncogenes and tumor suppressor genes in different sites of head and neck squamous cell. *Anti-cancer Res* 1998; 18:4793-800.

Teman S, Kawaguchi H, El-Naggar AK, Jelinek J, Tang H, Liu DD, Lang W, Issa JP, Lee JJ, Mao L. Epidermal growth factor receptor copy number alterations correlate with poor clinical outcome in patients with head and neck squamous cancer. *J Clin Oncol* 2007; 25:2164-70.

Todd R, Hinds PW, Munger K, Rustgi AK, Opitz OG, Suliman Y, Wong DT. Cell cycle dysregulation in oral cancer. *Crit Rev Oral Biol Med* 2002; 13:51-61.

Tomashefski JF Jr, Connors AF Jr, Rosenthal ES, Hsiue IL.Peripheral vs central squamous cell carcinoma of the lung. A comparison of clincial features, histopathology, and survival. *Arch Pathol Lab Med* 1990; 114:468-74.

Travis WD, Colby TV, Corrin B, Shimosato Y, Brambilla E. *Histological Typing of Lung and Pleural Tumours.* Sobin LH. Series ed. World Health Organization. International Classification of Tumours. Berlin, Heidelberg, New York: Springer-Verlag, 1999.

Ueda G, Sunakawa H, Nakamori K, Shinya T, Tsuhako W, Tamura Y, Kosugi T, Sato N, Ogi K, Hiratsuka H. Aberrant expression of beta- and gamma-catenin is an independent prognostic marker in oral squamous cell carcinoma. *Int J Oral Maxillofac Surg* 2006; 35:356-61.

Uematsu K, He B, You L, Xu Z, McCormick F, Jablons DM. Activation of the Wnt pathway in non- small cell lung cancer: evidence of dishevelled overexpression. *Oncogene* 2003; 22:7218-21.

Vogelstein B, Kinzler KW. The multi-step nature of cancer. *Trands Genet* 1993; 9:138-41.

Wang Z, Shu W, Lu MM, Morrisey EE. Wnt7b activates canonical signaling in epithelial and vascular smooth muscle cells through interaction with Fzd1, Fzd10, and LRP5. *Mol Cell Biol* 2005; 25:5022-30.

Weinberg RA. The retinoblastoima protein and cell cycle control. *Cell* 1995; 81:323-30.

Wiencke JK. DNA adduct burden and tobacco carcinogenesis. Oncogene 2002; 21:7376-91.

Willert K, Nusse R. Beta-catenin; a key mediator of Wnt signaling. *Curr Opin Genet Dev* 1998; 8:95-102.

Wistuba II, Behrens C, Milchgrub S, Bryant D, Hung J, Minna JD, Gazdar AF. Sequential molecular abnormalities are involved in the multi-stage development of squaemous cell lung carcinoma. *Oncogene* 1999; 18:643-50.

Wistuba II, Behrens C, Virmani AK, Mele G, Milchgrub S, Girad L, Fondon JW 3rd, Garner HR, McKay B, Latif F, Lerman MI, Lam S, Gazdar AF, Minna JD. High resolution chromosome 3p allelotyping of human lung cancer and pre-neoplastic/pre-invasive bronchial epithelium reveals multiple, discontinuous sites of 3p allele loss and three regions of frequent breakpoints. *Cancer Res* 2000; 60:11949-60.

Worsham MJ, Chen KM, Meduri V, Nygren AO, Errami A, Schouten JP, Benninger MS. Epigenetic events of disease progression in head and neck squamous cell carcinoma. *Arch Otolaryngol Head Neck Surg* 2006; 132:668-77.

Xu J, Gimenez-Conti IB, Cunningham JE, Collet AM, Luna MA, Lanfranchi HE, Spitz MR, Conti CJ. Alterations of p53, cyclin D1, Rb, and H-ras in human oral carcinomas related to tobacco use. *Cancer* 1998; 83:204-12.

In: Squamous Cell Carcinoma   ISBN: 978-1-61209-929-3
Editor: Daniel V. Mortensen   © 2012 Nova Science Publishers, Inc.

Chapter 3

REGULATION OF CELL PROLIFERATION IN ORAL SQUAMOUS CELL CARCINOMA

Marcelo Donizetti Chaves[1], Mariza Akemi Matsumoto[2],
Patrícia Pinto Saraiva[2], and Daniel Araki Ribeiro[1]
[1]Centro de Ciências Sociais, Saúde e Tecnologia,
Universidade Federal do Maranhão, MA, Brazil
[2]Departamento de Ciências da Saúde,
Universidade do Sagrado Coração, USC, Sao Paulo, Brazil
[3]Departmento de Biociências,
Universidade Federal de São Paulo, UNIFESP, Sao Paulo, Brazil

ABSTRACT

Oral squamous cell carcinoma is the most common head and neck cancer and it often has a poor prognosis, owing to local tumor invasion and frequent lymph node metastasis. The development of oral squamous cell carcinoma is usually preceded by a premalignant phase, the most common of which is leukoplakia. Mechanisms of oncogenesis are intimately linked to cell proliferation disruption recognized by intense division and growth, and disturbed maturation. However, for a number of reasons, squamous cell carcinoma is advanced detected, usually when malignant transformation occurred, once it was proved to present specific gene mutation associated. Preceding oral cancer phase, some potentially malignant disorders can appear, marked by alterations in cell kinetics. Herein, the present chapter aims to review the regulation of cell proliferation in development of oral squamous cell carcinoma. Such information plays an important role for understanding the disease, as well as the importance of the detection of preceding oral lesions.

1. INTRODUCTION

Cancers of the head and neck region (oral cavity, pharynx, and larynx) are the sixth most common malignancy worldwide (1). Involving the oral cavity account for 2–3% of all malignancies (2). The tumors are different origins but to squamous cell carcinoma, which represents approximately 90% to 95% of cancer cases in mouth (3,4) and the others 10% are cancers types diagnosed non-squamous cell carcinomas, sarcomas, lymphomas, and melanomas.

The oral squamous cell carcinoma (OSCC) is defined as a malignant neoplasm derived from squamous epithelium, which can affect both the oral cavity (oral mucosa, gingiva, hard palate, tongue, and floor of the mouth) and the lip vermilion (5).

There is a geographic variation in the incidence of cancer of the head and neck among different countries of the world and among different regions within a country (6). Your prevalence indicates that the socio-cultural lifestyles of a population play an important role in oral carcinogenesis (7). Moreover its distribution and occurrence varies by age, ethnic group, and level of country development (8,9,10,11)

According the American Cancer Society in 2009 the USA had 23,110 new cases of cancer of the oral cavity and 5,370 deaths (10) In European Union this numbers in the same year is 39, 833 new cases of oral cancer and 13,634 deaths. (12) In Asia, 80% of head and neck cancers are usually found in the oral cavity and oropharynx (13,14).

The oral cancer is among the 10 most common types of malignancies in the Brazilian population. According to the National Cancer Institute (INCA), this type of carcinoma is the fifth highest incidence in men (with an estimated 10,330 cases) and the seventh most frequent type of cancer in women (with an estimated 3,790 cases) (15).

It has been suggested that the cancer has increased in several countries such as Australia, Sweden, India and central and eastern European countries (13,14). In contrast, the incidence of oral oropharyngeal cancer is decreasing in some areas of Latin America (16, 17).

2. CAUSES

This attributable to the combined effect of ageing, and high or increasing levels of the prevalence of cancer risk factors such as tobacco, unhealthy diet, physical inactivity and infections (18).

The etiology of OSCC is strongly associated with tobacco and alcohol consumption (19, 20). From relative risk factors of alcohol and tobacco, it has been estimated, that 75% of all oral cancers are preventable. In the remaining 25% of patients who are not exposed to these substances, the cause/s of their tumors remains unknown (21).

Many constituents of tobacco smoke are carcinogenic and thus able to induce mutations in the genetic material or pro-carcinogens that during metabolism induce the formation of harmful substances. Alcohol is also considered a risk factor because the products of its metabolism, especially acetaldehyde producers of free radicals that cause mutations in DNA. (22)

Not only the use of tobacco but also the act of chewing betel mainly in India and Southeast Asia has been strongly associated with an increased risk for oral cancer. (23,24)

Ultraviolet radiation is also included in the list of risk factors that induction of SCC, especially the lower lip, where it may occur by the DNA damage (25)

Another risk factor is human papillomavirus (HPV), which is also associated with benign and malignant oral lesions (59% HPV positivity). (26). The prevalence of HPV in OSCC is extremely diverse, ranging from 0% to 100% in the literature, and the prevalence of HPV in other head nek cancer iis not uncommon (27, 28, 29)

Among those, only HPV subtypes 16,18 proceed to malignant transformation (27,30) but the tumorigenic conversion requires the presence of other risk factors.(29)

In several epidemiological studies the importance of diet and nutrition in oral neoplasia has been indicated (31). Fruits and vegetables (high in vitamins A and C) are described as protective in oral cancer and precancer. (32)

Another factors has been associated with increased the risk for development of carcinoma of the oral cavity as iron deficiency anemia in Plummer-Vinson or Paterson-Kelly syndrome) (33), increase age (34) immunosuppression, immunosuppressive medications and sistemic diseases. (35).

Factors most controversial such as chronic irritation from dental factors too has been proposed (36,37,38).

3. INCIDENCE

Men are affected twice as often as women probably due to increased exposure to these risk factors. (39) In some cases as in Taiwan this ratio can reveal a male predominance of 15:1 (40) .However, this difference in male and female ratio is becoming less pronounced, probably because women have been more equally exposing themselves to known oral carcinogens such as tobacco and alcohol.(41,42)

Most patients are older than 45 years of age (39), being rare in young patients where approximately 4–6% of oral cancer occurs in patients aged less than 40 years. Recently it has been observed that there is an increasing incidence of OSCC in the younger population of several countries. (43)

Clinical presentation of these early OSCC is usually in the form asymptomatic of a white lesion (leukoplakia), red lesion (erythroplakia), or a mixed of both (erythroleukoplakia) may mimic other conditions. (44)

The leukoplakia appears as a slightly elevated grayish-white plaque develop surface irregularities (granular or nodular leukoplakias), papillary surface (verrucous or verruciform leukoplakia) (44) with uncommom multifocal involvement (proliferative verrucous leukoplakia) (45)

Presents frequency of dysplastic or malignant alterations in oral leukoplakia has ranged from 15.6 to 39.2 percent in several studies. (46)

The floor of mouth was the most common site, with (42.9% of leukoplakias showing some degree of dysplasia, carcinoma in situ, or invasive OSCC followed by tongue (24.2%) and lip (24.0%) also sites with dysplasia or carcinoma present. (47, 48)

Already erythroplasia although less common than leukoplakia, it is much more likely to show dysplasia or carcinoma. Fifty-one percent showed invasive, 40% with severe epithelial dysplasia or carcinoma in situ and 9% mild-to-moderate dysplasia (49)

Red lesions are asymptomatic, atrophic, and inflammatory, with or without white areas (50, 51). The areas greatest involvement are floor of mouth, lateral tongue, retromolar pad, and soft palate are the most common sites.(44) Is this phase that there is little or no symptoms and innocuous

appearance of the lesion can often delay the diagnosis and treatment of OSCC
(52)

When analyzed all forms of lesions the incidence of oral cancer by
primary location varies depending on the geographic region. Some reports
have noted the tongue was the most common site, followed, in order of
decreasing frequency, by the floor of the mouth, palate, and gingiva (alveolar
ridge) (7,53), while others note the predominance of lesions in the floor of the
mouth (30%), followed by the tongue (28%) and the lower lip (13%), (48)

In advanced stages the OSCC presented ulceration of the mucosal surface,
bleeding, induration and exophytic growth (54). Other lesions have an
endophytic growth with a depressed, surface invagination, rounded border
(49).

These forms the OSCC should be distinguished from other malignancies
such as lymphoma, metastases and sarcomas. In the early stages of the
malignancy an incorrect clinical diagnosis is more likely to be made (55)

Symptoms include pain (56) and mobility of teeth, problems in breathing,
difficulty in speech, dysphagia, trismus, and paraesthesia (57) are observed in
more advanced cases. Skin fistulas, severe anaemia and cachexia are found in
terminal patients. Cervical lymphadenopathy may be present with or without
any other symptoms. (58)

About 5%, a cervical lymph node enlargement is detected in the absence
of any obvious primary tumour (59).

Other lesions are defined by the use of betel quid chewing that often
results progressive, scarring lesions of the mouth known as oral submucous
fibrosis that showed a malignant transformation rate of 7.6 percent for oral
submucous fibrosis. (60)

Some studies have suggested that clinical presence of oral lichen planus,
especially the erosive form, may be associated with an increased cancer risk,
although other investigators have questioned the strength of this
association.(61,62)

4. DIAGNOSIS

Typical clinical features of OSCC are found in advanced stages making
easy to determine the diagnosis but one must always take a biopsy to confirm
the histopatology diagnosis (63)

Histopatologically diagnosis is based on the degree of cell differentiation and distribute in three categories according to the WHO as well, poor and moderately differentiated. (64)

The first, tissue architecture is similar to the pattern of normal squamous epithelium. The poorly differentiated exhibit a predominance of immature cells, numerous typical and atypical mitoses and minimal keratinization. The moderately differentiated exhibit some degree of nuclear pleomorphism, little mitotic activity and keratinization (64) but as many authors no founded correlation between the histopathology classification and prognostic value (65,66) the WHO suggests that others factors should be added to histopathology as the pattern of invasion and lymph node conditions (67).

The tumor (size and the presence of deep muscle or bone invasion), node, metastasis (TNM) staging of intraoral tumors has been used for this purpose and usually provides a reliable basis for estimation of therapeutic planning and still remains the important tool for the clinician in predicting disease outcome. It seems particularly useful in the prediction of prognosis of later stage cancers (68).

The observation of these items show that OSCC has a relatively unfavorable prognosis (69) with a 5-year survival of 35%-50% (70). The presence of affected lymph node is strongly associated with a decreased survival to approximately 50% (71). Therefore the T and N stage have been shown to be excellent prognostic markers but they cannot predict the tumor's biologic properties.

The TNM stages III and IV showed to poor prognosis in patients with OSCC (72). The same patients with bilateral metastases of the cervical nodule have poorer prognosis than those with unilateral metastasis (73). TNM stages III and IV are more closely related to the presence of neural infiltration and lymphatic embolization, thus showing that patients with clinical stage IV have lower survival time (54), whereas, those with TNM I and II are disease free after 5 year follow-up (74).

The presence of tumor positive lymph nodes is reportedly a weighty prognostic factor in OSCC, but the high propensity for occult locoregional metastases (20-45%) (75,76) is the important disadvantage for the use of clinical staging, particularly in early stage OSCC (T1/T2N0) (77).

Metastases from OSCC most frequently affected the ipsilateral cervical lymph nodes. For tumors of the base of tongue the main region of the lymph node metastasis is contralateral or bilateral cervical. From the floor of mouth and lower lip may initially develop in the submental nodes. If there is perforation of the capsule that covers the nodule by the tumor with consequent subsequent invasion of adjacent connective tissue the node will feel fixed and immovable. In 30% of cases of oral cancers during the clinical evaluation there is a palpable or occult cervical metastasis complicating diagnosis (78).

More recently, many workers have used genetically based methods for molecular (gene expression profiling) signatures to predict cervical lymph node metastasis in OSCC. The identification of quantifiable variables of molecular level, which directly or indirectly condition the tumor biology, could help the clinician to determine the state of risk of a patient and thereby select the best therapeutic options (79).

The incidence of distant metastasis from OSCC regions varies from 5 to 24% in clinical reports (80) and is higher than 40% in some autopsy examinations (81).

Distant metastases are most common in the lungs, bone and hepatic (metastases occur less commonly), but any part of the body may be affected. (44, 82)

The OSCC shows a strong tendency to recur, and its recurrence is associated with a poor prognosis for survival. Recurrence is particularly prominent in SCC of the tongue and floor of mouth (83).

5. TREATMENT

A possible treatment strategy for these tumors could be a more aggressive initial approach combining several treatment modalities.

The form of treatment depending on the location and extension of the primary tumor, TNM stage of disease and general health of the patient. maybe only surgical, exclusively through radiotherapy, or a combination of both (84).

Early dysplastic lesions sometimes may be reversible if the source of injury can be eliminated. Lesions showing moderate epithelial dysplasia should be removed or destroyed if possible. (44)

For advanced-stage disease, surgery with adjuvant radiation therapy may be indicated. The particular surgical approach is influenced by site, location, size, depth of infiltration and proximity to bone. Tumours that involve the jaw require marginal mandibulectomy and mandibulotomy. In metastases from OSCC cervical lymphadenectomy has played an important role in the management (85).

Radiotherapy plays a key role in the management of early-stage and locally advanced OSCC (86).

In some cases chemotherapy may become an important adjunctive role although not a curative approach. It is usually used adjunctively or palliatively in cases of very large, unresectable lesions or distant metastasis. (87, 88).

6. REGULATION OF CELL PROLIFERATION IN ORAL CARCINOGENESIS

Nowadays, the proportion of cells committed to the cycle may be easily assessed by Ki-67 or MIB-1 antibodies, which identify an antigen expressed in G1, S and G2 phases of cycling cells (89). In addition, PCNA is a DNA polymerase delta auxiliary protein of 36KDa, which is closely related to the replication of DNA and is indispensable to cell proliferation. PCNA level increases rapidly in mid-G1, remains elevated throughout the S phase, and then decreases from G2/M to G1 (90). PCNA-positive cells can be regarded as cells involved in the proliferating process. A decrease in the PCNA-positive cells reflects a decrease in S phase and, thus, a reduced proliferative activity. Detection of PCNA antigen is considered a reliable marker of cell proliferation (91). Previous studies conducted by our group have revealed that PCNA positive nuclei were higher either in oral dysplasia or in squamous cell carcinomas when compared to ordinary oral mucosa (92). These results suggest that the expression of PCNA is closely involved during neoplastic conversion.

Retinoblastoma (Rb) and p16 gene products are part of the retinoblastoma pathway that negatively controls the cell cycle. The Rb gene is located on the long arm of chromosome 13. The retinoblastoma protein is a nuclear phosphoprotein that is expressed in most normal cells. Rb functions during the G1–S transition within the cell cycle (93). The hypophosphorylated form of the retinoblastoma protein mediates G1 arrest (93). Rb and p16 genes inactivation have been reported in many cancers (94). Cyclin-dependent kinase inhibitors (CDKIs), such as p21 exert a direct control on the cell cycle. p21 is a negative regulators of cyclin-dependent kinases and in this function they are negative check-point regulators of the cell cycle. Some studies have suggested that p21 in carcinoma of oral cavity seems to be predictive parameter in regulation and prognosis of squamous cell carcinomas (95). Cellular DNA damage leads via p53-activation to an up-regulation of p21 to cause cell-cycle arrest in the G1 phase with the cellular possibility for DNA-repair or the induction of apoptosis (96). In addition, p21 can be regulated independent of p53 by cellular growth factors (97). Particularly, our results have demonstrated no significant statistically differences (p>0.05) in expression of all tumor suppressor genes along medium-term oral carcinogenesis assay (98).

Dysregulation of the cell cycle in cancer cells can also be due to inactivation of critical CKIs or to overexpression of cyclins. For example, the inhibition of the CKI p16, generally by hypermethylation of its promoters, leads to loss of function and has been associated with various malignancies such as melanoma, lung, breast and colorectal tumors (99). Therefore, the goal in cancer therapy was the development artificial CKI targeted to CDKs. Such agents are pan-cyclin-dependent kinase (CDK) inhibitor (e.g., Flavopiridol) resulting in cell cycle arrest, with consequent arrest of the uncontrolled grow, and induction of apoptotic cell death by inhibition of antiapoptotic molecule including bcl-2 (99). This is because no mutations in the p16CDKN2A exon 2 were found in any experimental periods evaluated that corresponded to normal oral mucosa, hyperplasia, dysplasia and squamous cell carcinomas following oral carcinogenssis induced by 4NQO (100). However, the levels of Rb were increased (p<0.05) in pre-neoplastic lesions at 12 weeks following carcinogen exposure. In well-differentiated squamous cell carcinoma induced after 20 weeks of treatment with carcinogen, p16 and Rb were expressed in some tumor cells (98). Taken together, our results support the notion that expression of Rb is closely event related to malignant transformation and conversion of the oral mucosa, being reliable biomarker linked to oral cancer pathogenesis.

It has been proposed that in many tumors the G1 phase is a frequent primary target, since most, if not all, human cancers show a dysregulated control of G1 progression where the major targets are exactly the Rb and p53 pathways, which contain several targets (Rb, p53, CDKs, cyclins) often altered (101). Treating such tumors by trying to kill these mutated cells with DNA-damaging agents such as ionizing radiation and DNA-targeting drugs, results in the cell checkpoint-mediated arrest at S or G2. Such remaining checkpoint can be used by the tumor cells to protect themselves from the radiation or cytotoxic agents. The situation may be tackled by associating the ionizing radiation or DNA-damaging drugs with inhibitors of S or G2 checkpoints, forcing the cancer cells carrying DNA lesions to enter mitosis, prompting a mitotic catastrophe and associated cell death. So, abrogation of DNA-damage checkpoint in S or G2 is a strategy for selectively targeting G1-checkpoint defective cancer cells (102). Normally, wild-type p53 has a very short half-life on the order of 6-20 min, and, therefore, it cannot be detected by standard immunohistochemical methods. Therefore, positive staining for p53 has been proposed as an indicator of mutations within the *Tp53* gene (103). In addition, regulatory defects of the *Tp53* gene may, in some cases, result in the over-expression or stabilization of the wild-type p53 protein. In an earlier study performed by our research group, an increased number of faintly or densely stained p53-positive cells, which were either wild-type and/or mutant, were found in the epithelium of dysplastic lesions and squamous cell carcinoma when compared to ordinary oral mucosa (104).

Bcl-2 and bax are also two important effector genes responsible for arresting cell cycle as a result of triggering the apoptosis process. The bcl-2 proto-oncogene was originally discovered by analysis of the t(14;18) chromosomal translocation associated with human follicular B-cell lymphoma (105). The bcl-2 gene encodes a protein located in the nuclear membrane, on the inner surface of mitochondria, and the endoplasmic reticulum. It is the most important gene of the bcl-2 family and has been shown to be an inhibitor of apoptosis (105). Immunohistochemical overexpression of bcl-2 has been observed in carcinomas of the nasopharynx, lung, urinary bladder, colon, prostate, breast, thyroid and oral cavity (106). Bax, another member of the bcl-2 family, is considered to be a major effector of apoptosis (107). In normal and tumour tissues, the distribution of bax is inversely related to that of bcl-2 (107). Thus, the bcl-2/bax ratio controls the relative susceptibility of cells to lethal stimuli (107). Our data pointed out an overexpression of bcl-2 and bax ($p < 0.01$) in all layers of the rat oral 'normal' epithelium exposed to chemical carcinogen during 4 weeks (108). The expression levels were the same in all layers of epithelium for both the antibodies used (bcl-2 or bax). In dysplastic lesions at 12 weeks following carcinogen administration, the levels of bcl-2 and bax expression did not increase when compared to negative control with the immunoreactivity for bcl-2 being restricted to the superficial layer of epithelium (108). In well-differentiated squamous cell carcinoma induced after 20 weeks of treatment with neoplasm inducer, bcl-2 was expressed in some cells of tumour islands. On the other hand, immunostaining for bax was widely observed at the tumour nests. The labeling index for bcl-2 and bax showed an increase ($P < 0.05$) after only 4 weeks (108). In conclusion, our results suggest that abnormalities in the apoptosis pathways are associated with the development of persistent clones of mutated epithelial cells in the oral mucosa. Bcl-2 and bax expression appears to be associated with a risk factor in the progression of oral cancer.

In mammals, apoptosis is mainly modulated by two protein families, the bcl-2 and inhibitor of apoptosis (IAP) proteins (109). Among IAP proteins, interest has been addressed to survivin, a multifunctional protein that suppresses apoptosis by association with caspases and Smac/DIABLO and regulates mitosis by interacting with other chromosomal passenger proteins (109). Unlike other IAP proteins broadly expressed in adult cells, survivin is expressed during embryonic development, and is not detectable in most differentiated normal adult tissues (109). Survivin is expressed in a wide variety of human malignancies, apparently as a requirement for cancer-cell immortalization and/or malignant progression (109). Although no histopathological abnormalities were induced in the oral epithelium of Wistar rats after 4 weeks of carcinogen exposure, survivin was expressed in some cells of the 'normal' oral epithelium (98). In pre-neoplastic lesions at 12 weeks following carcinogen exposure, the levels of survivin were increased ($p < 0.05$) when compared to negative control. In well-differentiated squamous cell carcinoma induced after 20 weeks of treatment with chemical carcinogen, survivin was expressed in some tumor cells (98). Lack of immunoreactivity for both markers was observed in the negative control group. Taken together, it seems that expression of survivin is considered an early event during malignant transformation and conversion of the oral mucosa.

REFERENCES

[1]   Rautava J, Luukkaa M, Heikinheimo K et al. Squamous cell carcinomas arising from different types of oral epithelia differ in their tumor and patient characteristics and survival. *Oral Oncol* 2007; 43(9): 911–9.

[2]   Alazawi W, Pett M, Arch B et al. Changes in cervical keratinocyte gene expression associated with integration of human papillomavirus 16. *Cancer Res* 2002; 62: 6959–6965

[3]   von Dongen GA, Snow GB. Prospectives for future studies in head and neck cancer. *Eur J Surg Oncol* 1997; 23: 485–91.

[4]   Landis SH, Murray T, Bolden S, Wingo PA, Cancer statistics, 1999. *CA Cancer J Clin* 1999; 49: 8-31.

[5]   Jordan RC, Daley T. Oral squamous cell carcinoma: new insights. *J Can Dent Assoc* 1997; 63:517-25.

[6]   Hakulinen T, Andersen B, Pukkala E et al. Trends in cancer incidence in the Nordic countries. *Acta Pathol Microbiol Immunol Scand* 1986; 94:30–7.

[7]   Zain RB. Cultural and dietary risk factors of oral cancer and precancer— a brief overview. *Oral Oncol* 2001; 37: 205–210.

[8]   Petersen PE, Bourgeois D, Ogawa H et al. The global burden of oral diseases and risks to oral health. *Bull World Health Organ* 2005; 83: 661– 9.

[9]   Bosetti C, Malvezzi M, Chatenoud L et al. Trends in cancer mortality in the Americas,1970–2000. *Ann Oncol* 2005; 16: 489–511.

[10] Jermal A, Siegel R, Ward D et al. Cancer statistics, 2009. *CA Cancer J Clin* 2009; 59(4):225-249.

[11] Zini A, Czerninski R, Sgan-Cohen HD. Oral cancer over four decades: epidemiology, trends, histology, and survival by anatomical sites. *J Oral Pathol Med* 2010; 39: 299–305.

[12] International Agency for Research on Cancer (IARC). *GLOBOCAN* Section of Cancer Information Lyon, France: IARC, 2008.

[13] International Agency for Research on Cancer (IARC). Tobacco Habits Other Than Smoking: Betel-Quid and Areca-Nut Chewing and Some Related Nitrosamines. *IARC Monographs on the Evaluation of the Carcinogenic Risks to Humans.* Lyon, France: IARC, 1985.

[14] Parkin DM, Pisani P, Ferlay J. Estimates of the worldwide incidence of 25 major cancers in 1990. *Int J Cancer* 1999; 80(6): 827– 841.

[15] Brazil. Ministry of Health National Cancer Institute. *Estimate 2010: cancer incidence in Brazil / National Cancer Institute. - Rio de Janeiro: INCA,* 2009.

[16] Wunsch-Filho V. The epidemiology of oral and pharynx cancer in Brazil. *Oral Oncol* 2002;38:737–46.

[17] Franceschi S, Bidoli E, Herrero R, et al. Comparison of cancers of the oral cavity and pharynx worldwide: etiological clues. *Oral Oncol* 2000;36:106–15.

[18] Petersen PE. The World Oral Health Report 2003: continuous improvement of oral health in the 21st century – the approach of the WHO Global Oral Health Programme. *Community Dent Oral Epidemiol* 2003; 31(Suppl. 1): 3–23

[19] 19 - Bundgaard T, Wildt J, Frydenberg M, et al. Case control study of squamous cell cancer of the oral cavity in Denmark. *Cancer Causes Control* 1995; 6:57-67.

[20] Batista AC, Costa NL, Oton-Leite AF, et al. Distinctive clinical and microscopic features of squamous cell carcinoma of oral cavity and lip. Oral Surg Oral Med Oral Pathol Oral Radiol Endod 2010;109: 74-79.

[21] Walker DM, Boey G, McDonald LA. The pathology of oral cancer. *Pathology* 2003; 35:376-83.

[22] Sculy C, FieldJK, Tanzawa H . Genetic aberrations in oral or head and neck squamous cell carcinoma: 1. Carcinogen metabolism, DNA repair and cell cycle control – *Oral Oncology* 2000; 36:256-263.

[23] Pindborg JJ, Murti PR, Bhonsle RB, et al. Oral submucous fibrosis as a precancerous condition.*Scand J Dent Res* 1984; 92:224-229..

[24] Murti PR, Bhonsle RB, Gupta PC, et al.Etiology of oral submucous fibrosis with special reference to the role of areca nut chewing. *J Oral Pathol Med* 1995; 24:145-152.

[25] Kulms D, Zeise E, Poeppelmann B, Schwarz T. DNA damage, death receptor activation and reactive oxygen species contribute to ultraviolet radiation-induced apoptosis in an essential and independent way. *Oncogene* 2002;21(38):5844-5851.

[26] Gillison ML, Koch WM, Capone RB et al . Evidence for a causal association between human papillomavirus and a subset of head and neck cancers. *J Natl Cancer Inst* 2000; 92:709-20.

[27] Gillison ML, Shah KV. Human papillomavirus- associated head and neck squamous cell carcinoma: mounting evidence for an etiologic role for human papillomavirus in a subset of head and neck cancers. *Curr Opin Oncol* 2001: 13: 183–188.

[28] Syrjanen S. Human papillomavirus (HPV) in head and neck cancer. *J Clin Virol* 2005; 32: 59–66.

[29] Lee SY, Cho NH, Choi EC et al: Relevance of human papilloma virus (HPV) infection to carcinogenesis of oral tongue cancer. *Int. J. Oral Maxillofac. Surg.* 2010; 39: 678–683.

[30] Scully C. Oral squamous cell carcinoma; From a hypothesis about a virus, to concern about possible sexual transmission. *Oral Oncol* 2002; 38:227-34.

[31] De Stefani E, Deneo-Pellegrini H, Mendilaharsu M, Ronco A. Diet and risk of cancer of the upper aerodigestive tract. Foods. *Oral Oncol* 1999; 35:17-21.

[32] Negri E, Franceschi S, Bosetti C, Levi F et al. Selected micronutrients and oral and pharyngeal cancer. *Int J Cancer* 2000; 86:122-7.

[33] Larsson LG, Sandström A, Westling P. Relationship of Plummer-Vinson disease to cancer of the upper alimentary tract in Sweden. *Cancer Res* 1975; 35:3308-3316.

[34] Horner MJ, Ries LAG, Krapcho M, et al. *SEER Cancer Statistics Review*, 1975-2006. Bethesda, Md.: National Cancer Institute; 2009.

[35] de Visscher JG, Bouwes Bavinck JN, van der Waal I. Squamous cell carcinoma of the lower lip in renal-transplant recipients. Report of six cases. *Int J Oral Maxillofac Surg* 1997; 26:120-123.

[36] Thumfart W, Weidenbecher M, Waller G, Pesch HJ. Chronic mechanical trauma in the aetiology of oropharyngeal carcinoma. *J Maxillofac Surg* 1978; 6: 217–21.

[37] Warnakulasuriya S. Causes of oral cancer-an appraisal of controversies. *Br Dent J* 2009; 207: 471–5.

[38] Piemonte ED, Lazos JP, Brunotto M Relationship between chronic trauma of the oral mucosa, oral potentially malignant disorders and oral cancer *J Oral Pathol Med* 2010;39: 513–517.

[39] Krolls SO, Hoffman S: Squamous cell carcinoma of the oral soft tissues: A statistical analysis of 14,253 cases by age, sex and race. *J Am Dent Assoc* 1976; 92:571.

[40] Ahmed F, Islam KM. Site predilection of oral cancer and its correlation with chewing and smoking habit—a study of 103 cases. *Bangladesh Med Res Counc Bull* 1990;16: 17–25.

[41] Silverman S Jr. Epidemiology. In: Silverman S Jr ed. *Oral Cancer*. 4th ed. Hamilton, Ontario, Canada: BC Decker Inc;1998;1-6.

[42] Chen JK, Katz RV, Krutchkoff DJ. Intraoral squamous cell carcinoma. Epidemiologic patterns in Connecticut from 1935 to 1985. *Cancer* 1990;66: 1288-1296.

[43] McLaughlin JK, Gridley G, Block G.Dietary factors in oral and pharyngeal cancer. *J Natl Cancer Inst* 1988: 80: 1237–1243

[44] Neville BW, Day, TA. Oral Cancer and Precancerous Lesions CA Cancer *J Clin* 2002;52:195-215

[45] Hansen LS, Olson JA, Silverman S Jr. Proliferative verrucous leukoplakia. A long-term study of thirty patients. *Oral Surg Oral Med Oral Pathol* 1985;60:285-298.

[46] Feller L, Altini M, Slabbert H. Pre-malignant lesions of the oral mucosa in a South African sample: A clinicopathologic study. *J Dent Assoc South Africa* 1991;46:261-265.

[47] Waldron CA, Shafer WG. Leukoplakia revisited: A clinicopathologic study of 3256 oral leukoplakias. *Cancer* 1975;36:1386-1392.

[48] Ribeiro ACP, Silva ARS, Simonato LE et al. Clinical and histopathological analysis of oral squamous cell carcinoma in young people A descriptive study in Brazilians *British Journal of Oral and Maxillofacial Surgery* 2009;47:95–98

[49] Mashberg A, Samit A. Early diagnosis of asymptomatic oral and oropharyngeal squamous cancers. CA *Cancer J Clin* 1995;45:328-351.
[50] Mashberg A: Erythroplasia vs. leukoplakia in the diagnosis of early asymptomatic oral squamous carcinoma. *N Engl J Med* 1977;297:109-110.
[51] Mashberg A, Merletti F, Boffetta P, et al: Appearance, site of occurrence, and physical and clinical characteristics of oral carcinoma in Torino - Italy. *Cancer* 1989;63:2522-2527.
[52] Kowalski LP, Carvalho AL, Martins Priante AV, Magrin J. Predictive factors for distant metastasis from oral and oropharyngeal squamous cell carcinoma. *Oral Oncol* 2005; 41(5): 534-41.
[53] Langdon JD. Epidemiology and aetiology. In: Henk JM, Langdon JD, eds. Malignant Tumors of the Oral Cavity. London: Edward Arnold, 18 1-208. 1985; 1-13.
[54] Bagan J, Sarrion G, Jimenez Y. *Oral cancer: Clinical features Oral Oncology* 2010; 46:414–417.
[55] Silverman S. *Oral cancer. Semin Dermatol* 1994;13:132–7.
[56] Sato J, Yamazaki Y, Satoh A et al. Pain is associated with an endophytic cancer growth pattern in patients with oral squamous cell carcinoma before treatment *Odontology* 2010;98:60–64.
[57] Haya-Fernández MC, Bagán JV, Murillo-Cortés J, et al. The prevalence of oral leukoplakia in 138 patients with oral squamous cell carcinoma. *Oral Dis* 2004;10(6):346–8.
[58] Antoniades DZ, Styanidis K, Papanayotou P, Trigonidis G. Squamous cell carcinoma of the lips in a northern Greek population. Evaluation of prognostic factors on 5-year survival rate. *Eur J Cancer B Oral Oncol* 1995;31:333-9.
[59] Erdem F. Characterization of 3 oral squamous cell carcinoma cell lines with different invasion and/or metastatic potentials J Oral Maxill Surg 2006; 64(9): 24
[60] Murti PR, Bhonsle RB, Pindborg JJ, et al. Malignant transformation rate in oral submucous fibrosis over a 17-year period. *Community Dent Oral Epidemiol* 1985;13:340-341.
[61] Barnard NA, Scully C, Eveson JW, et al. Oral cancer development in patients with oral lichen planus. *J Oral Pathol Med* 1993;22:421-424.
[62] Eisenberg E. Oral lichen planus: A benign lesion. *J Oral Maxillofac Surg* 2000;58:1278- 1285.
[63] Silverman Jr S. Early diagnosis of oral cancer. *Cancer* 1988;62:1796–9.

[64] Barnes L, Eveson, JW, Reichart P, Sidransky D. World Health Organization Classification of Tumours. *Pathology andGenetics of Head and Neck Tumours.* Lyon: IARC Press; 2005.

[65] Anneroth G, Hansen LS, Silverman S Jr: Malignancy grading in oral squamous cell carcinoma. I. Squamous cell carcinoma of the tongue and floor of mouth: Histologic grading in the clinical evaluation. *J Oral Path* 1986; 15:162.

[66] Willen R, Nathanson A, Moberger G, et al: Squamous cell carcinoma of the gingiva: Histological classification and grading of malignancy. *Acta Otolaryngol* 1975;79:146.

[67] Barnes L, Eveson JW, Reichert P, Sidransky D. World Health Organization *Classification of Tumours. Pathology and Genetics of Head and Neck Tumours.* Lyon: IARC Press; 2005.

[68] Kantola S, Parikka M, Jokinen K, et al. Prognostic factors in tongue cancer – relative importance of demographic, clinical and histopathological factors. *Brit J Cancer* 2000;83(5):614–9.

[69] Platz H, Fries R, Hudec M, et al. The prognostic relevance of various factors at the time of the first admission of the patient. *J Maxillofac Surg* 1983;11:3-12

[70] Wildt J, Bjerrum P. Squamous cell carcinoma of the oral cavity: a retrospective analysis of treatment and prognosis. *Clin Otolaryngol* 1989;14:107-13.

[71] Preuss SF, Dinh V, Klussmann JP, Semrau R, Mueller RP, Guntinas-Lichius O. Outcome of multimodal treatment for oropharyngeal carcinoma: a single institution experience. *Oral Oncol* 2007; 43(4): 402-7.

[72] Nicolson IGL. Tumor oncogene expression and the metastatic phenotype. *Cancer* 2000;3(4):25-57.

[73] Kerdpon D, Sriplung H. Factors related to advanced stage oral squamous cell carcinoma in southern Thailand. *Oral Oncol.* 2001; 37 (3):216-21.

[74] Araújo Júnior RF, Costa A de LL, Ramos CCF. Clinical- pathological parameters as prognostic indicators in oral squamous cell. *Pesq Bras Odontoped Clin Integr.* 2006; 6 (2):125-30.

[75] Mendelson BC, Woods JE, Beahrs OH. Neck dissection in the treatment of carcinoma of the anterior two-thirds of the tongue. *Surg Gynecol Obstet* 1976;143:75-80.

[76] Kremen AJ. Results of surgical treatment of cancer of the tongue. *Surgery* 1956;39:49-53.

[77] Yoshida K, Kashima K, Suenaga S, et al. Immunohistochemical detection of cervical lymph node micrometastases from T2N0 tongue cancer. *Acta Otolaryngol* 2005;125(6):654–8.

[78] Shah JP, Candela FC, Poddar AK.The patterns of cervical lymph node metastasis from squamous carcinoma of the oral cavity. *Cancer* 1990;66:109-113

[79] Roepman P, Wessels LF, Kettelarij N, et al. An expression profile for diagnosis of lymph node metastases from primary head and neck squamous cell carcinomas. *Nat Genet* 2005;37(2):182–6.

[80] Merino OR, Lindberg RD, Fletcher GH. An analysis of distant metastases from squamous cell carcinoma of the upper respiratory and digestive tracts. *Cancer* 1977;40:145–151.

[81] Zbaren P, Lehmann W. Frequency and sites of distant metastases in head and neck squamous cell carcinoma. An analysis of 101 cases at autopsy. *Archives of Otolaryngology, Head & Neck Surgery* 1987;113:762–764.

[82] Calhoun KH, Fulmer P, Weiss R, Hokanson JA. Distant metastases from head and neck squamous cell carcinomas. *Laryngoscope* 1994;104:1199–1205.

[83] Lehman RH, Cox JD, Belson TP, et al. Recurrence patterns by treatment modality of carcinomas of the floor of the mouth and oral tongue. *Am J Otolaryngol* 1982;3:174- 181.

[84] Giannini A, Ninu MB, Gallina E. Parametri istopatologici e metastatizzazione linfonodale nel carcinoma laringeo sopraglottico. *Patológica* 1991;83:167-75.

[85] Pagedar NA, Gilbert RW. Selective neck dissection: a review of the evidence. *Oral Oncol* 2009;45(4–5):416–20.

[86] Mazeron R, Tao Y, Lusinchi A, Bourhis J. Current concepts inmanagement in head and neck cancer; radiotherapy. *Oral Oncol* 2009;45(4–5): 402–8.

[87] Licitra L, Grandi C, Guzzo M, et al. Primary chemotherapy in resectable oral cavity squamous cell cancer: A randomized controlled trial. *Journal of Clinical Oncology* 2003;21:327–333.

[88] Vokes EE, Stenson K, Rosen FR, et al. Weekly carboplatin and paclitaxel followed by concomitant paclitaxel, fluorouracil, and hydroxyurea chemoradiotherapy: Curative and organ-preserving therapy for advanced head and neck cancer. *Journal of Clinical Oncology* 2003;21:320–326.

[89] Catoretti G, Becker MHG, Key G. Monoclonal antibodies agains recombinant parts of the Ki-67 antigen (MIB-1 and MIB-3) detect

proliferating cells in microwave-processed formalin-fixed paraffin sections *J Pathol* 1992;168:357-363

[90] Linden MD, Torrex RX, Dubus J, Zarbo RJ. Clinical application of morphologic and immunocytochemical assessments of cell proliferation [editorial] *Am J Clin Pathol* 1992;97: S4-13

[91] Tanaka T, Kohno H, Sakata Y, Yamada Y, Hirose Y, Sugie S, Mori H. Modifying effects of dietary capsaicin and rotenone on 4-nitroquinoline 1-oxide-induced rat tongue carcinogenesis *Carcinogenesis* 2002;23: 1361-1367

[92] Silva RN, Ribeiro DA, Salvadori DM, Marques ME Placental glutathione S-transferase correlates with cellular proliferation during rat tongue carcinogenesis induced by 4-nitroquinoline 1-oxide Exp Toxicol Pathol 2007;59:61-8.

[93] Muirhead DM, Hoffman HT, Robinson RA.Correlation of clinicopathological features with immunohistochemical expression of cell cycle regulatory proteins p16 and retinoblastoma: distinct association with keratinisation and differentiation in oral cavity squamous cell carcinoma J Clin Pathol 2006;59:711-715.

[94] Nemes JA, Deli L, Nemes Z, Márton IJ. Expression of p16(INK4A), p53, and Rb proteins are independent from the presence of human papillomavirus genes in oral squamous cell carcinoma *Oral Surg Oral Med Oral Pathol Oral Radiol Endod* 2006;102:344-352

[95] Goto M, Tsukamoto T, Inada K, Mizoshita T, Ogawa T, Terada A, Hyodo I, Shimozato K, Hasegawa Y, Tatematsu M. Loss of p21WAF1/CIP1 expression in invasive fronts of oral tongue squamous cell carcinomas is correlated with tumor progression and poor prognosis *Oncol Rep* 2005;14:837-846

[96] Hill R, Bodzak E, Blough MD, Lee PW. p53 binding to the p21 promoter is dependent on the nature of DNA damage Cell Cycle 2008;15:2535-2543

[97] Ciccarelli C, Marampon F, Scoglio A, Mauro A, Giacinti C, De Cesaris P, Zani BM. p21WAF1 expression induced by MEK/ERK pathway activation or inhibition correlates with growth arrest, myogenic differentiation and onco-phenotype reversal in rhabdomyosarcoma cells Mol Cancer 2005;4:41-46.

[98] Ribeiro DA, Kitakawa D, Domingues MA, Cabral LA, Marques ME, Salvadori DM Survivin and inducible nitric oxide synthase production during 4NQO-induced rat tongue carcinogenesis: a possible relationship Exp Mol Pathol 2007;83:131-7

[99] Schwartz GK and Shah M.A. Targeting the Cell Cycle: A New Approach to Cancer Therapy. *J Clin Oncol* 2005;23:9408-9421.

[100] Minicucci EM, da Silva GN, Ribeiro DA, Favero Salvadori DM No mutations found in exon 2 of gene p16CDKN2A during rat tongue carcinogenesis induced by 4-nitroquinoline-1-oxide J Mol Histol 2009;40:71-6a

[101] Dela Val B, and Birnbaun, D. A cell cycle hypothesis of cooperative oncogenesis. *International Journal Of Oncology* 2007;30: 1051-1058

[102] Lapenna, S. and Giordano, A. Cell cycle kinases as therapeutic targets for cancer. *Nature Reviews Drug Discovery* 2009;8:547-566

[103] Okazaki Y, Tanaka Y, Tonogi M and Yamane G. Investigation of environmental factors for diagnosing malignant potential in oral epithelial dysplasia *Oral Oncol* 38: 562-573, 2002

[104] MInicucci EM, Ribeiro DA, Silva GN, Pardini ME, Mantovani JC, Salvadori DM. The role of TP53 gene during rat tongue carcinogenesis induced by 4-nitroquinoline 1-oxide, *Exp Toxicol Pathol*, 2009b, *in press*

[105] 105 - Tsujimoto Y, Jaffe E, Cossman J, Gorham J, Nowell PC, Croce CM. Clustering of breakpoints on chromosome 11 in human B-cell neoplasms with the t(11;14) chromosome translocation *Nature* 1985;315, 340–343

[106] Singh BB, Chandler FW Jr, Whitaker SB, Forbes-Nelson AE. Immunohistochemical evaluation of bcl-2 oncoprotein in oral dysplasia and carcinoma Oral Surg Oral Med Oral Pathol Oral Radiol Endod 1998;85, 692–698.

[107] Oltvai ZN, Milliman CL, Korsmeyer SJ. Bcl-2 heterodimerizes in vivo with a conserved homolog, Bax, that accelerates programmed cell death *Cell* 1993;74, 609–619.

[108] Ribeiro DA, Salvadori DM, Marques ME Abnormal expression of bcl-2 and bax in rat tongue mucosa during the development of squamous cell carcinoma induced by 4-nitroquinoline 1-oxide *Int J Exp Pathol* 2005;86:375-81

[109] Altieri DC, Survivin, versatile modulation of cell division and apoptosis in cancer, *Oncogene* 2003;22:8581–8589

In: Squamous Cell Carcinoma
Editor: Daniel V. Mortensen

ISBN: 978-1-61209-929-3
© 2012 Nova Science Publishers, Inc.

Chapter 4

SQUAMOUS CELL CARCINOMA ARISING IN EPIDERMAL CYST AND HUMAN PAPILLOMAVIRUS ASSOCIATED CYST

Teresa Pusiol
Institute of Anatomic Pathology, Rovereto Hospital,
Rovereto (TN), Italy

ABSTRACT

The squamous cell carcinoma (SCC) arising in epidermal cyst (EC) is a very rare malignant disease but is an enigmatic pathological event and it's hard to find in human pathology a malignancy so surprising and so easy to diagnose. Human papillomavirus associated cyst (HPAC) is a type of epithelial cyst with microscopic features consistent with human papillomavirus (HPV) infection. Only HPV 57 and 60 has been identified in the cystic wall to date. These HPV types are often associated with malignant diseases (high-risk HPV). In this chapter, we describe three cases of SCC arising in epidermal cyst (EC) and the first case of SCC arising in HPAC. Serial sections of all specimens had been prepared in order to verify that the cystic appearance was real and not merely the result of poor orientation of the specimen. In all cases, sections of paraffin-embedded tissue were investigated for the presence of HPV-DNA sequences by polymerase chain reaction (PCR) and *in situ* hybridization. In the first case, an 88-year-old man presented a right zigomatic mass. Histopathology revealed a cyst lined by squamous epithelium in continuity with invasive keratinizing SCC. In the second case, a 96-year-old man consulted your Hospital regard to 1.5x1cm nodule of the right ear's helix. Histopathology showed the typical cystic wall of an EC with transition to invasive keratinizing SCC. In the third case, a 67 year-old man showed ulcerated nodular cystic lesion of the right helix, of 8mm in maximum diameter. Histologically a cystic lesion was lined by squamous epithelium in continuity with invasive SCC. Finally an 86 years-old woman suffered of a perineal cystic nodule of 1.5cm in diameter. Histologically the cystic lesion showed the wall with varying degrees of papillomatosis, hypergranulosis, parakeratosis with dysplastic and koilocytic changes. Areas of *in situ* and invasive SCC were found. Human HPV 16 was detected. Computed tomography with the administration of intravenous contrast material was performed and showed diffuse wall thickening of the anorectum and infiltration of anus muscles'levator. *Endoscopic biopsies* of *the anal* canal and *rectum* revealed SCC with presence of HPV 16. The patient refused every treatment. Malignant degeneration of EC may be diagnosed only with the support of an accurate histopathological documentation in order to exclude mimics (proliferating epidermal cyst, proliferating trichilemmal cyst). Regarding HPAC, the site, the malignant transformation and the finding of HPV 16 type, may be considered features of an extraordinary rare case.

INTRODUCTION

A cyst (C) is an enclosed space within a tissue, usually containing fluid and lined by epithelium. The Cs are usually classified on the basis of their pathogenesis. The most important cutaneous Cs are derived from the dermal appendages, as retention Cs. The appendageal Cs include: epidermal C, HPV – related C, proliferating epidermal C, trichilemmal C, proliferating trichilemmal C, hybrid C, hair matrix C, pigmented follicular C, cutaneous keratocyst, vellus hair C, steatocystoma multiplex, milium, eccrine hidrocystoma, and apocrine hidrocystoma. The squamous cell carcinoma (SCC) arising in epidermal C is a very rare malignant disease, an enigmatic pathological event, and it's hard to find a so surprising and so easy to diagnose malignancy in human pathology. Human papillomavirus-associated cyst (HPAC) is a type of epithelial C with microscopic features consistent with human papillomavirus (HPV). To date, cases of SCC arising in HPAC have not been reported. We described three cases of SCC arising in epidermal Cs and the first report of SCC arising in HPAC with emphasis to diagnostic criteria in order to establish accurate diagnosis.

MATERIALS AND METHODS

An amount of 4 SCC arising in cutaneous Cs were was examined: three cases in epidermal C and a case in HPAC. The medical records for each case were reviewed and the following attributes were recorded: age, sex, duration and location. The lesions were fixed in phosphate-buffered formalin and embedded in paraffin. Sections were stained with haematoxylin-eosin. Serial sections of all specimens had been prepared in order to verify that the cystic appearance was real and not merely the result of poor orientation of the specimen. In all cases sections of paraffin-embedded tissue were investigated for the presence of HPV-DNA sequences by polymerase chain reaction (PCR) and in situ hybridization.

RESULTS

Squamous cCell cCarcinoma aArising in eEpidermal cCyst

Table 1 reported the clinico-pathological features of the squamous cell carcinomaSCC arising in epidermal cCyst.

Table 1. Clinico-pathological features of the squamous cell carcinoma arising in epidermal cyst neoplasms

Nr.	Age/sex	Clinical presentation	Treatment	Macroscopic features	Follow up
1	88/man	Right zigomatic area	Tumorectomy	Cystic mass of 7 mm. in maximum diameter	Free of disease 28 months after tumorectomy
2	96/man	Nodular lesion of the right helix	Tumorectomy	Cystic tumour of 1.6x1x1 cm	Free of disease 18 months after tumorectomy
3	67/man	Ulcerated nodular lesion of the right helix	Tumorectomy	Cystic mass of 8 mm. in maximum diameter	Free of disease 12 months after tumorectomy

In all cases, histopathological examination revealed a cyst lined by stratified squamous epithelium exhibiting keratinization. The cystic epithelium showed *in situ* SCC in continuity with invasive keratinizing component. PCR and in situ hybridization for HPV research were negative. A diagnosis of invasive SCC arising in the wall of an epidermal C was performed (Figures 1,2,3,4,5).

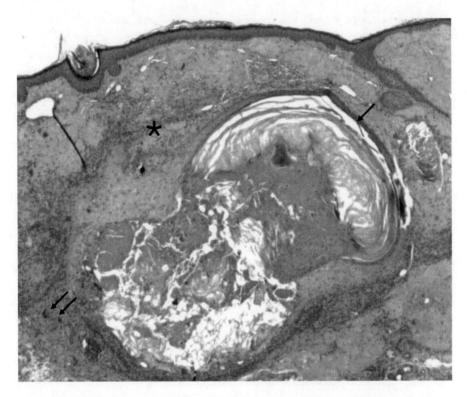

Figure 1. Squamous cell carcinoma arising in epidermal cyst (Case 1). The histological section show typical epidermal cyst, lined by a stratified squamous epithelium with granular cell layer (arrow). The epithelium showed dysplastic area in continuity with carcinoma (star). Granulomatous inflammation is evident corresponding to cystic parietal rupture (double arrow). The cystic lumen contains keratin fragments (H&E;40x).

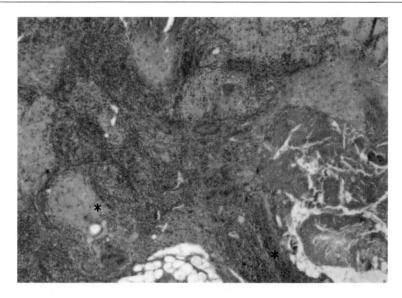

Figure 2. Squamous cell carcinoma arising in epidermal cyst (Case 1). Squamous cell carcinoma is found in the dermis and in continuity with cystic epithelium (stars). Granulomatous inflammation is with multinucleated cells reactive to keratin is evident (H&E; 100x).

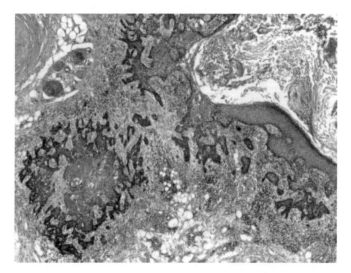

Figure 3. Squamous cell carcinoma arising in epidermal cyst (Case 2). The cyst wall is composed of a benign stratified squamous epithelium with transition to squamous cell carcinoma (H&E; 25x).

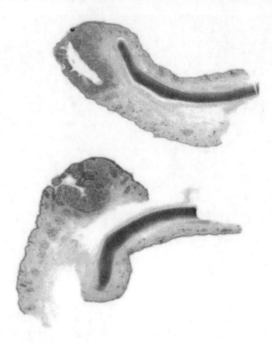

Figure 4. Squamous cell carcinoma arising in epidermal cyst (Case 3). The macroscopic illustration show cystic cutaneous lesions and helix cartilage.

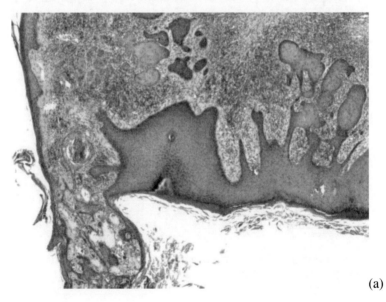

(a)

Figure 5. (continued on next page).

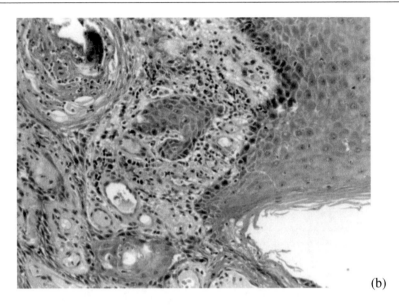

(b)

Figure 5. A: Squamous cell carcinoma arising in epidermal cyst (Case 3). The cystic epithelium show acanthosis, hyperkeratosis, dysplastic change and is in continuity with carcinomatous proliferations. (H&E;40x). B: At high magnification the squamous carcinomatous proliferation is evident (H&E; 100x).

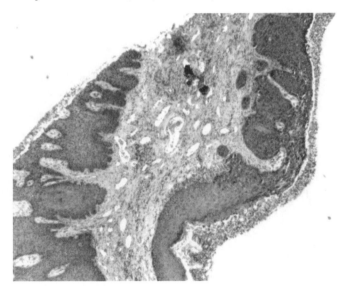

Figure 6. Squamous cell carcinoma arising in human papillomavirus associated cyst (Case 4). *In situ* and invasive squamous carcinomatous areas are evident in continuity with cystic wall (H&E; 40X).

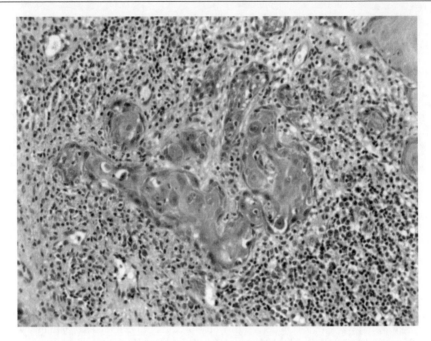

Figure 7. Squamous cell carcinoma arising in human papillomavirus associated cyst (Case 4). The invasive squamous carcinomatous component is in continuity is evident (H&E; 100X).

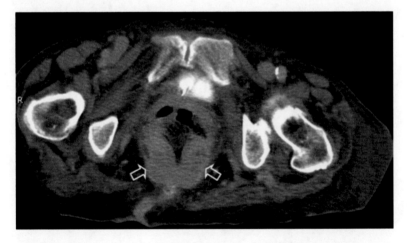

Figure 8. Squamous cell carcinoma arising in human papillomavirus associated cyst (Case 4). Enhanced CT scan of the pelvis shows diffuse wall thickening of the anorectum and infiltration of anus levator's muscle (arrows). No enlarged pelvic lymph nodes were revealed.

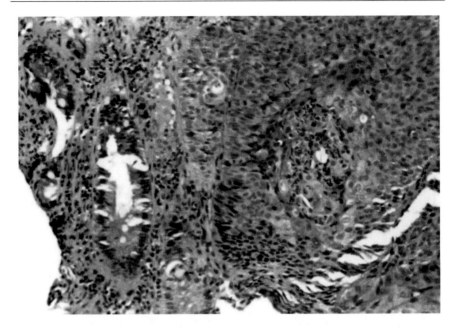

Figure 9. Infiltration by squamous cell carcinoma of rectal mucosa is evident (H&E; 100X).

DISCUSSION

Among the various types of appendageal Cs SCC has been reported to arise from proliferating trichilemmal C, proliferating epidermal C, and epidermal C.

Proliferating trichilemmal C may exhibit marked cytologic atypia and a worrisome number of mitoses [1]. Therefore, it was suggested that a diagnosis of carcinomatous transformation of a proliferating trichilemmal C should only be made in the presence of infiltrative margins, high mitotic activity (4 to 5 x high-power field) or metastases [2].

Based on this approach, Lopez-Rios et al. [3] found 30 well-documented cases of so-called malignant proliferating trichilemmal Cs (malignant proliferating trichilemmal tumour, giant hair matrix tumour, trichochlamydocarcinoma) published in the English literature.

Ackermann et al. believe that a proliferating trichilemmal C (pilar tumour) is a variant of squamous-cell carcinoma. They use the term "proliferating trichilemmal C squamous-cell carcinoma "for such cases [4-5]. This view has not yet received wide acceptance. [6]

Sau P. et al. have studied 33 proliferating epidermal Cs and found carcinomatous changes in seven cases. [7]

We believe that proliferating epidermal C is a neoplasm, not a C.

Epidermal Cs are common on face, neck and trunk but can occur in virtually any anatomic location. These lesions are usually located in the mid and lower dermis but they do not shell out like the tricholemmal C. There is often a surface punctum. Epidermal Cs are sometimes associated with other anomalies, such as nevus comedonicus or the Favre-Racouchot syndrome. They are also a cutaneous manifestation of Gardner's syndrome. It is likely that some epidermal Cs constitute a developmental anomaly of the follicular infundibulum, although in other instances traumatic implantation is probably also a cause (producing the "epidermal inclusion C) [8], particular on the palms and soles [9] and in the subungual region [10].

Epidermal C are lined by squamous epithelium showing epidermal keratinization, that is, the formation of keratohyaline granules and flattened surface epithelium. Several histological variations in the epidermal lining have been reported. These include focal epidermal proliferation, [11], a seborrheic keratosis-like change, [12], basal hyperpigmentation (seen in black patients) [13], melanophagic proliferation [14], focal pilomatrixoma-like changes (usually in kindreds with Gardner's syndrome [15 - 16 – 17], clear cell change [18] cornoid lamellation [19], epidermolytic hyperkeratosis [20], histological changes of Darier's disease [20,21], pyogenic granuloma formation [22,12], Paget's disease, [23],basal cell carcinoma [24],[19] mycosis fungoides, and Bowen's disease [22,25].

Cases of malignant transformation of epidermal C reported in older literature, have been questioned as some; at least some cases may represent proliferating trichilemmal Cs or proliferating epidermal Cs. 16 cases of SCC arising in EC have been reported to date (Table 2) [2326, 2427, 2528, 2629, 2730, 2831, 2932, 3033, 3134, 3235, 3336, 3437, 3538, 3639]. Lopez Rios et al [3033] reviewed 27 cases reported in the English literature. These authors identified only 7 cases in which microscopic description and adequate figures corresponded to "SCC arising in a cutaneous epidermal cyst". On the other hand Miller's [2528] and Yaffe's [2629] cases had not complete histopathological illustrations. Some considerations could be made about this small series because it includes some curious cases. The 21-year-old woman reported by Morgan et al [3336] is the youngest patient with cutaneous SCC described in the literature. The case reported by Debaize et al [3437], with a size of 20cm and a weight of 1.535g, is the biggest one described in the literature.

A lesion may be diagnosed as "SCC arising in an EC" only with the support of an accurate histopathological documentation in order to exclude mimics (proliferating epidermoid cyst, proliferating trichilemmal cyst and pseudocarcinomatous hyperplasia in a ruptured cyst). Serial sections of all specimens had been prepared in order to verify that the cystic appearance was real and not merely the result of poor orientation of the specimen. HPV demonstration has to be negative in order to exclude a HPAC. The main histological feature essential for diagnosis is the presence of a "continuum" between cystic wall and squamous cell carcinoma proliferation. Applying this diagnostic criterion many reported cases shouldn't been classified in this group. In your series, two cases of SCC arising in epidermal C were localized in the helix. SCC of the external ear comprises one fourth of all squamous cell cutaneous carcinomas of the head and neck region [5659] . most patients are elderly. The tumors are more common in the auricle (particularly the helix) than in the canal [5760,5861,5962]. The pattern of local spread varies depending on the initial location of the tumor, a finding that also applies to basal cell carcinomas. Tumors of the helix spread initially along the helix and then before to the antihelix and after to the posterior surface of the ear; tumors of the antihelix spread concentrically; tumors of the posterior surface of the ear spread to the helix and along that structure [6063]. The prognosis is much better for tumors of the auricle than for those in the canal, a fact that is at least partially related to the earlier diagnosis of the former type of tumor [6063,6164].

In 1982, Meyer et al [3942] described 5 cases of "verrucous cysts", in which they detected HPV genomes by polymerase chain reaction (PCR), without specifying HPV type. The specific HPV type in HPAC was not been identified until 1992, when Matsukura et al [4043] cloned HPV type from a cyst that showed non homology with other known prototypes of HPV (from HPV 1 through HPV 59), so that it was named HPV 60. In 1998, Egawa K et al [41] (44) detected HPV 57 DNA by PCR and ISH in the plantar cyst of a 23-years old Japanese man. HPACs most commonly arise in the palmoplantar region [4245, 4346, 4447], although similar lesions have been reported on the scalp [4548], face [4649, 4750], neck [4750], trunk [4144, 4548, 4750], arm [4144, 4750], and leg [4750]. HPACs have been described adjacent to warty lesions [4144, 4851, 4952] in patients after organ transplantation. HPV infection is associated with a broad spectrum of human diseases, ranging from subclinical lesions to benign and malignant conditions [5053, 5154]. HPV 6 and 11 are usually associated with benign diseases (low risk HPV) [5053-5154]. HPV 16 and 18 and, to some extent 33 and 31, are often associated with malignant diseases (high-risk HPV) [5053, 5154]. Our case is the first description documenting the presence of HPV 16 in HPAC [4144, 5255]. P16^{INK4a} is commonly expressed in cervical dysplasias and carcinomas associated with high risk HPV. Confirmation of high grade squamous intraepithelial abnormality is provided by the so-called "block-positivity", i.e. immunoreactivity involving every cell in the complete, or almost complete, thickness of the squamous neoplastic epithelium [5356]. In our case p16^{INK4a} immunostaining showed diffuse and intense positivity throughout the cystic epithelium and in the areas of invasive SCC confirming the presence of a high risk HPV in the cystic wall and in the invasive SCC. To our knowledge the present case is the first description of SCC arising from HPAC in the literature, with involvement of adjacent organ.

Anal cancer is a slowly progressing disease that begins as a superficial mass and may spread locally, involve regional lymph nodes or metastasize to distant organs [5457]. Approximately 72% of invasive anal cancer cases are associated with HPV 16 and/or 18 infections. This estimate of 16 HPV and 18 prevalence is similar to the found in invasive cervical cancer cases [5558].

The pathogenesis of a simultaneous HPV infection of both anal canal and HPAC is unclear. The modality of C infection by HPV is not known. Two hypotheses may exist: 1. the epidermis infected by HPV could have been implanted into the dermis; 2. HPV could initially have infected the upper part of eccrine duct, such as the acrosyringeal epithelium and then could have migrated into various parts of the dermal portions of the eccrine duct, where the virus-associated epidermoid cysts developed. The eccrine duct was not evident because of neoplastic destruction. A previous sexual contact could be responsible for anal infection by HPV 16, considering that carcinogenetic effect of infection may have a long latency period. In conclusion, SCC arising in HPAC, HPV type, patient's age, coexistence of HPV-related SCCs in anorectum and perineal HPAC cyst are features of an extraordinary rare case of human pathology.

Table 2. Squamous cell carcinoma arising in cutaneous epidermal cysts: review of the literature

Authors	Age/Sex	Site	Duration of lesion	Size of cyst (cm)	Treatment	Outcome
Davidson et al. (1976)	52 M	L frontal region	2 months	NS	Excision	Free of disease
Bauer et al. (1980)	68 M	R retroauricular area	4 months	3	Excision + parotidecto my	Free of disease
Miller et al. (1981)	34 M	L retroauricular area	NS	8	Excision + RT 5,325 R	Free of disease after 25 years
Yaffe et al. (1982)	58 M	R ear	11 years	2.5	Excision	Free of disease
Arianayaga m et al. (1987)	59 F	L tight	3 months	7	Excision + inguinal dissection	Lymph node metastasis; died after 6 months
Shah et al. (1989)	55 F	L gluteal region	6 months	10	Excision	NS
Davies et al. (1994)	32 M	L index finger	10 years	NS	Amputatio n + RT	Free of disease
López-Ríos et al. (1999)	66 M	L retroauricular area	2 months	1.5	Excision	Free of disease
Malone et al. (1999)	92 F	R forehead	NS	NS	Excision	No recurrence after 10 months
Wong et al. (2000)	57 NS	L buttock	20 years	6	Excision	Free of disease after 6 months
Morgan et al. (2001)	5 cases, 21-80 (mean age 56,7) 3 M, 2 F	Face, Neck, Trunk.	NS	NS	Excision	Free of disease (mean follow-up 2-6 years)
Debaize et al. (2002)	38 F[1]	L buttock area	Since adolescence	20x15	Excision	Free of disease after 1 year
Cameron et al. (2003)	67 M	R temple	3 months	3	Excision	Free of disease after 6 months
Chiu et al. (2007)	74 M	Prossimal L thigh	40 years	15	Excision	Free of disease after 2 years

NS: not stated; RT: radiotherapy; L: left; R: right; M: male; F: female; SCC: squamous cell carcinoma.

---

[1] Not invasive

REFERENCES

[1]   Swanson PE, Marrogi AJ, Wick MR. Histologic characterization of pilar carcinoma as distinct from proliferating pilar tumor (abstract*).* L Cutan Pathol 1990; 17:320

[2]   Amaral AL, Nascimento AG, Goellner JR. Proliferating pilar (trichilemmal) cysts. Report of two cases, one with carcinomatous transformation and one with distant metastases. *Arch Pathol Lab Med* 1984;108:808-10

[3]   López-Ríos F, Rodríguez-Peralto JL, Aguilar A, Hernández L, Gallego M. *Am J Dermatopathol.* 2000;2:183-7

[4]   Noto G. "Bening" proliferating trichilemmal tumour: does it really exist? *Histopathology* 1999;35:386-387

[5]   Mones JM, Achermann AB. Proliferating trichilemmal cyst is squamous-cell carcinoma. *Dermatopathology: Practical & Conceptual* 1988;4:295-310

[6]   G, Pravati G, Aricò M. Proliferating trichilemmal cyst should always be considered as a low-grade carcinoma. *Dermatology* 1997;194:374-375.

[7]   Sau P, Graham JH, Helwig EB. Proliferating epithelial cysts. Clinicopathological analysis of 96 cases. *J Cutan Pathol.* 1995;22:394-406

[8]   Greer KE. Epidermal inclusion cyst of the sole. *Arch Dermatol.* 1974;109:251-2

[9]   (Fisher BK, Macpherson M. Epidermoid cyst of the sole. *J Am Acad Dermatol.* 1986;15:1127-9

[10] (Yung CW, Estes SA. Subungual epidermal cyst. *J Am Acad Dermatol.* 1980;3:599-601

[11] Vicente J, Vazquez-Doval FJ. Proliferations of the epidermoid cyst wall. *Int J Dermatol* 1998; 37:181-185

[12] Rahbari H. Epidermoid cysts with seborrheic verruca-like cyst walls. Arc Dermatol 1982;118:326-328

[13] Fieselman DW, Reed RJ; Ichinose H: Pigmented epidermal cyst. *J Cutan Pathol* 1974; 1:256-259

[14] Vaideeswar P, Prabhat DP, Sivaraman A. Epidermal inclusion cyst with melanoma-like melanophagic proliferation. *Acta Derm Venereol* 1999; 79:88

[15] Narisawa Y, Kohda H. Cutaneous cysts of Gardner's syndrome are similar to follicular stem cells. *J Cutan Pathol* 1995;22:115-121

[16] (Cooper PH, Fechner RE. Pilomatricoma-like changes in the epidermal cysts of Gardner's syndrome. *J Am Acad Dermatol* 1983;8:639-644

[17] (Leppard BJ, Bussey HJR. Gardner's syndrome with epidermoid cysts showing features of pilomatrixomas. *Clin Exp Dermatol* 1976;1:75-82

[18] Satoh T, Mitho Y, katsumata M et al. Follicular cyst derived from hair matrix and outer root sheath. *J Cutan Pathol* 1989; 16: 106-108

[19] Vicente J, Vazquez-Doval FJ. Proliferations of the epidermoid cyst wall. *Int J Dermatol* 1998;37:181-185

[20] Vicente J, Vazquez-Doval FJ. Proliferations of the epidermoid cyst wall. *Int J Dermatol* 1998;37:181-185

[21] Mittag H. Darier's disease involving an epidermoid cyst. *J Cutan Pathol* 1990; 17:388-390

[22] Hunt SJ. Two pyogenic granulomas arising in an epidermoid cyst. *Am J Dermatopathol.* 1989;11:360-3

[23] Vicente J, Vazquez-Doval FJ. Proliferations of the epidermoid cyst wall. *Int J Dermatol* 1998;37:181-185

[24] Vicente J, Vazquez-Doval FJ. Proliferations of the epidermoid cyst wall. *Int J Dermatol* 1998;37:181-185

[25] Shelley WB, Wood MG. Occult Bowen's disease in keratinous cysts. *Br J Dermatol* 1981;105:105-108.

[26] Davidson TM, Bone RC, Kiessling PJ. Epidermoid carcinoma arising from within an epidermoid inclusion cyst. *Ann. Otol. Rhinol. Laryngol..* 1976;85: 417-8.

[27] Bauer BS, Lewis VL. Carcinoma arising in sebaceous and epidermoid cysts. *Plast. Surg.* 1980:5;222-4.

[28] Miller JM. Squamous cell carcinoma arising in an epidermal cyst. *Arch. Dermatol.* 1981;117: 683.

[29] Yaffe HS. Squamous cell carcinoma arising in an epidermal cyst. *Arch. Dermatol.* 1982;118:961.

[30] Arianayagam S, Jayalakshmi P. Malignant epidermal cyst: a case report. *Mal. J. Pathol.* 1987;9:89-91.

[31] Shah LK, Rane SS, Holla VV. A case of squamous cell carcinoma arising in an epidermal cyst. *Indian J. Pathol. Microbiol.* 1989;32:138-140.

[32] Davies MS, Nicholson AG, Southern S, Moss AHL. Squamous cell carcinoma arising in a traumatically induced epidermal cyst. *Injury.* 1994;25:116-7.

[33] López-Ríos F, Rodríguez-Peralto JL, Castaño E, Benito A. Squamous cell carcinoma arising in a cutaneous epidermal cyst: case report and literature review. *Am. J. Dermatopathol.* 1999;21:174-7.

[34] Malone JC, Sonnier GB, Hughes AP, Hood AF. Poorly differentiated squamous cell carcinoma arising within an epidermoid cyst. *Int. J. Dermatol.* 1999;38:556-8.

[35] Wong TH, Khoo AK, Tan PH, Ong BH. Squamous cell carcinoma arising in a cutaneous epidermal cyst-a case report. *Ann. Acad. Med. Singapore.* 2000;29:757-9.

[36] Morgan MB, Stevens GL, Somach S, Tannenbaum M. Carcinoma arising in epidermoid cyst: a case series and aetiological investigation of human papillomavirus. *Br. J. Dermatol.* 145(2001)505-6.

[37] Debaize S, Gebhart M, Fourrez T, Rahier I, Baillon JM. Squamous cell carcinoma arising in a giant epidermal cyst: a case report. *Acta. Chir. Belg.* 2002;102:196-8.

[38] Cameron DS, Hilsinger RL Jr. Squamous cell carcinoma in an epidermal inclusion cyst: case report. *Otolaryngol Head Neck Surg.* 2003;129:141-3.

[39] Chiu MY, Ho ST. *Squamous cell carcinoma arising from an epidermal cyst.* Hong Kong Med. J. 2007;13: 482-4.

[40] Marjolin, L.N. *Ulcere in Dictionariee de Mèdicine.* 1828;21:31-50.

[41] Steffen C. "Marjolin's ulcer. Report of two cases and evidence that Marjolin did not describe cancer arising in scars of burns". *Am J Dermatopathology* 1984:187-93

[42] Meyer LM, Tyring SK, Little WP. Verrucous cyst. *Arch Dermatol.* 1991;127:1828-9.

[43] Matsukura T, Iwasaki T, Kawashima M. Molecular cloning of a novel human papillomavirus (type 60) from a plantar cyst with characteristic pathological changes. *Virology.* 1992;190:561-4.

[44] Egawa K, Kitasato H, Honda Y, Kawai S, Mizushima Y, Ono T. Human papillomavirus 57 identified in a plantar epidermoid cyst. *Br J Dermatol.* 1998;138:510-4.

[45] Egawa K, Inaba Y, Ono T, Arao T. 'Cystic papilloma' in humans? Demostration of humnan papillomavirus in plantar epidermoid cysts. *Arch Dermatol* 1990; 126: 1599-603.

[46] Egawa K, Honda Y, Inaba. Yet al Detection of human papillomaviruses and eccrine ducts in palmoplantar epidermoid cysts. *Br J Dermatol* 1995; 132: 533-42.

[47] Rios-Buceta LM, Fraga-Fernandez J, Femandez-Herrera J. Hurman. Papillomavirus in an epidermoid cyst of the sole in a non-Japanese patient. *J Am Acad Dermatol* 1992;27:364-6.

[48] Elston DM, Parker LU, Tuthill PJ. Epidermoid cyst of the scalp containing human papillomavirus. *J Cutan Pathol* 1993;20:184-6.

[49] Aloi F, Tornasini C, Pippione M. HPV-related follicular cysts. *Am J Dermatopathol* 1992;14:37-41.

[50] Soyer HP, Schadendorf D, Cerroni L, Kerl H. Verrucous cysts; Histopathologic characterization and molecular detection of human papillomavirus-specific DNA. *J Cutan Pathol* 1993;20:411-7.

[51] Jung K-D, Kim P-S, Lee J-H, et al. Human papillomavirus-associated recurrent plantar epidermal cysts in a patient after organ transplantation. *J Eur Acad Dermatol Venereol.* 2009;23:837-9.

[52] Egawa K, Egawa N, Honda Y. Human papillomavirus-associated plantar epidermoid cyst related to epidermoid metaplasia of the eccrine duct epithelium: a combined histological, immunohistochemical, DNA-DNA in situ hybridization and three-dimensional reconstruction analysis. *Br J Dermatol* 2005;152:961-967.

[53] McMurray HR, Nguyen D, Westbrook TF, McAnce Dl. Biology of human papillomaviruses. *Int J Exp Pathol.* 2001;82:15-33

[54] Nebesio CL, Mirowski GW, Chuang TY. Human papillomavirus: clinical significance and malignant potential. *Int J Dermatol.* 2001;40:373-9.

[55] Kitasato H, Egawa K, Honda Y, Ono T, Mizushima Y, Kawai S. A putative human papillomavirus type 57 new subtype isolated from plantar epidermoid cysts without intracytoplasmic inclusion bodies. *J Gen Virol.* 1998;79:1977-81.

[56] Mulvany NJ, Allen DG, Wilson SM. Diagnostic utility of p16INK4a: a reappraisal of its use in cervical biopsies. *Pathology.* 2008;40:335-44.

[57] Roach SC, Hulse PA, Moulding FJ et al Magnetic resonance imaging of anal cancer. *Clin Radiol* 2005;60:1111-1119.

[58] Smith JS, Lindsay L, Hoots B, et al. Human papillomavirus type distribution in invasive cervical cancer and high-grade cervical lesions: a meta-analysis update. *Int J Cancer* 2007;121:621-632.

[59] Avila J, Bosch A, Aristizabal S, Frìas Z, Marcial V. Carcinoma of the pinna. *Cancer* 1977, 40: 2891-95.

[60] Barnes L, Johnson JT. Clinical and pathological considerations in the evaluation of major head and neck specimens resected for cancer. *Part II Pathol Annu* 1986, 21:82-110.

[61] Lewis JS. Cancer of the ear. *CA Cancer J Clin* 1987, 37:78-87.
[62] Shiffman NJ. Squamous cell carcinomas of the skin of the pinna. *Can J Surg* 1975, 18:279-283.
[63] Bailin PL, Levine HL, Wood BG, Tucker HM. Cutaneous carcinoma of the auricular and periauricular region. *Arch Otolaryngol* 1980, 106: 692-696.
[64] Johns ME, Headington JT. Squamous cell carcinoma of the external auditory canal. A Clinicopathologic study of 20 cases. *Arch Otolarungol* 1974, 100:45-49.

In: Squamous Cell Carcinoma   ISBN: 978-1-61209-929-3
Editor: Daniel V. Mortensen   © 2012 Nova Science Publishers, Inc.

Chapter 5

EPIDERMOLYSIS BULLOSA AND
SQUAMOUS CELL CARCINOMA

Minhee Kim[2], Lizbeth RA Intong [1,2], and
*Dedee F Murrell[*1,2]*
[1]Department of Dermatology, St. George Hospital, Sydney, Australia
[2]The University of New South Wales, Sydney, Australia

FREQUENCY OF SCC DEVELOPMENT IN EB

Squamous cell carcinoma (SCC) in the context of epidermolysis bullosa (EB) is a life threatening complication known to arise at least once in 2.6% of all EB patients with varying degrees of frequency across different subtypes of EB [1]. To date, Fine and colleagues' study of 3280 EB patients from the National EB Registry (NEBR) in the United States over the 20-year period (1986-2006) remains the largest epidemiological study of EB [1]. According to the data from the NEBR, the frequency of SCC was highest in recessive dystrophic EB, generalized severe (RDEB-GS), followed by RDEB, generalized other (RDEB-O), junctional EB, Herlitz (JEB-H) and other subtypes of EB simplex (EBS) as summarized in Table-1. All subtypes of EBS

* Corresponding author: Professor Dedee F Murrell, MA, BM, FAAD, MD, FACD, Head,
  Department of Dermatology, St George Hospital, Sydney, University of NSW, Australia,
  Email: d.murrell@unsw.edu.au

and Dominant Dystrophic EB (DDEB) had the lowest frequency of SCC (<1%), reflecting the risk of SCC development similar to that of the general American population. All the SCC arising in EBS subtypes developed in sun-exposed areas, further suggesting that the pathogenesis of SCC in EBS is most likely related to significant ultraviolet exposure. In contrast, there is a significant increased risk of SCC development in JEB-H (4.4%), RDEB-O (9.6%) and RDEB-GS (22.7%). The majority of SCC especially in RDEB patients developed in chronic cutaneous wounds or cutaneous scars rather than sun-exposed areas, suggestive of a different carcinogenesis pathway unrelated to ultraviolet damage. One SCC case of non-cutaneous origin (tongue) has been observed in RDEB.

Table 1. Frequency of SCC in different subtypes of EB [1]

	Subtypes of EB					
	All EBS subtypes	JEB-H	JEB-nH	DDEB	RDEB-GS	RDEB-O
Total No. of patients	1669	45	191	422	141	280
No. of patients with SCC	4	2	1	3	32	27
Percentage	0.2	4.4	0.5	0.7	22.7	9.6

Abbreviations: DDEB, dominant dystrophic EB; EB, epidermolysis bullosa; EBS, EB simplex; JEB-H, Juctional EB, Herlitz; JEB-nH, junctional EB, non-Herlitz; RDEB-GS, recessive dystrophic EB, severe generalized; RDEB-O, recessive dystrophic EB, generalized other.

CUMULATIVE RISK OF SCC DEVELOPMENT AND DEATH FROM SCC IN EB

Development of SCC in all EBS subtypes with the exception of the one formerly called EBS-Koebner (EBS-K) appears to develop after the age of 65 with the cumulative risk well below 5% at the age of 65, which is a risk similar to that of the general American population [1]. Only one case of SCC was reported by Fine and colleagues for EBS-K in which the SCC arose at age 40 (cumulative risk = 3.8% by age 40). DDEB patients had a similarly low risk as EBS subtypes but the risk increased earlier with a cumulative risk of 1.5% by age 45, 4.5% by age 65 and 15% by age 75. JEB-H showed early increase, with a cumulative risk of 18.2% by age 25. Of more serious concern is the early and progressive rise of the cumulative risk of SCC development in RDEB-GS and RDEB-O (RDEB-nHS & RDEB-I; old RDEB classification) patients as summarized in Table-2. RDEB-GS had the highest cumulative risk and early development of SCC from ages over 15, rising to a peak of 90.1% by age 55. RDEB-O showed relatively slower and later rise in the cumulative risk of SCC development with moderately lower risk compared to RDEB-GS. Although the NEBR did not report any SCC in RDEB patients under the age 15, there have been cases of SCC development in RDEB patients as early as 6, 12 and 13 years of age and of many different ethnicities [2][3][4].

Table 2. Cumulative risk of SCC development in patients with RDEB subtypes [1]

Age	Cumulative Risk of SCC development		
	RDEB-GS	RDEB-nHS	RDEB-I
15	0	0.82	0
20	7.5	3.69	0
25	26.7	11.8	0
30	51.7	17.3	8.0
35	67.8	22.3	8.0
40	73.4	24.4	8.0
45	80.2	35.8	23.3
50	80.2	35.8	23.3
55	90.1	35.8	23.3

Abbreviations: RDEB-GS, recessive dystrophic epidermolysis bullosa, severe generalized; RDEB-I, recessive dystrophic epidermolysis bullosa, inversa; RDEB-nHS, recessive dystrophic epidermolysis bullosa, non-Hallopeau-Siemens.

CUMULATIVE RISK OF DEATH FROM SCC

The NEBR did not report any SCC related death in EBS, DDEB or JEB patients, however metastatic SCC was the most common cause of death in RDEB patients with RDEB-GS patients being at the highest risk of death at a much earlier age than RDEB-O (refer to Table-3). RDEB-GS patients with a history of SCC have a rapid rise of their risk of SCC-related death from ages 25 to 30, with the risk rising to 87.31% by age 45. RDEB, non-Hallopeau-Siemens (RDEB-nHS) and RDEB, inverse (RDEB-I) have much later increase in risk of SCC-related death, rising to 60% and 50% by age 55 respectively.

**Table 3. Cumulative risk of death from SCC in those
with a history of SCC [1]**

Age	Cumulative risk of death from SCC		
	RDEB-GS	RDEB-nHS	RDEB-I
15	0	3.9	0
20	12.7	3.9	0
25	19.2	11.9	0
30	42.3	16.3	0
35	57.2	30.6	0
40	81.0	30.6	0
45	87.3	37.2	50.0
50	87.3	37.2	50.0
55	87.3	60.05	50.0

Abbreviations: RDEB-GS, recessive dystrophic epidermolysis bullosa, severe generalized;
RDEB-I, recessive dystrophic epidermolysis bullosa, inversa; RDEB-nHS, recessive
dystrophic epidermolysis bullosa, non-Hallopeau-Siemens.

PATHOGENESIS OF SCCS IN RDEB

The pathogenesis appears to be mostly unrelated to ultraviolet exposure in RDEB as evident in the epidemiological and pathological characterization of SCC development in RDEB. As aforementioned, SCC in EBS mostly developed on sun-exposed areas whilst SCC in RDEB and JEB developed in chronic cutaneous ulcers and scars. Furthermore, the majority of RDEB patients develop more than one SCC, with a median of 3-3.5 and a range of 1-40 (Fine et al, 2009). The majority of SCC develops on bony prominences of the upper and lower extremities [5][6]. Histopathologically, the majority of RDEB related SCCs are well differentiated, however such cases often act aggressively and metastasize early. Thus, histological grade is a poor prognostic indicator in predicting tumor aggressiveness.

The severity and extent of ulceration and scarring of the skin seems to correlate with the risk of developing cutaneous SCC in EB sufferers [7]. Although there is a definitive lack of understanding in the pathogenesis of SCC in RDEB, several theories have been described to date. Goldberg's tissue stress theory hypothesized that ongoing tissue trauma in especially fragile skin and chronic ulceration may serve as a propagating factor for tissue carcinogenesis, as experimentally demonstrated in mouse studies by the implantation of a foreign body as a source of trauma [8]. The theory, however, fails to explain the mechanism initiating carcinogenesis in RDEB. According to Smoller and colleagues, only RDEB keratinocytes showed a premalignant potential when compared with keratinocytes cultured from EBS patients [9]. Immunohistochemical analysis for expression of filaggrin, involucrin, cytokeratins and the growth activation marker psi-3 of RDEB keratinocytes from previously healed ulcers for 2 years demonstrated evidence of a persistent growth-activated cell phenotype.

A few studies have described severe forms of EB as an immunodeficient state, which may contribute to the carcinogenesis of SCC. The natural killer cell activity in JEB, DDEB and RDEB was significantly decreased compared to normal controls, with RDEB exhibiting the most pronounced decrease [10]. Furthermore, significantly lower levels of lymphokines and monokines, specifically interferon-γ, interleukin-1 (IL-1) and IL-2, were present in RDEB and DDEB compared to healthy controls [11]. Thus, the lack of anti-tumor cellular immune activity, especially by natural killer cells and T-lymphocytes may have a contributory role in the carcinogenesis.

Arbiser and colleagues have demonstrated elevated levels of basic fibroblast growth factor (bFGF) levels in 51%, 13% and 0% of RDEB, EBS and JEB patients respectively [12]. Some of the roles of bFGF have been identified, and it serves as a potent angiogenic factor and a chronic stimulant for proliferation of keratinocytes. Furthermore, bFGF also stimulates the synthesis of collagenase. A study in transgenic mice has shown that increasing the collagenase activity increases the incidence of SCC in skin, most likely through direct tissue lysis and facilitation of tumor invasion [13]. Thus, bFGF and collagenase may have a significant role in tumorigenesis. With regards to facilitation of tumor invasion, RDEB associated SCC has been shown to overexpress matrix metalloproteinases 7 and 13 (MMP-7 & MMP-13), which may account for the aggressive and invasive nature of RDEB associated SCC [14].

Ortiz-Urda and colleagues have shown a significant role of the NC1 domain of collagen VII expression in precipitation of SCC in Ras-driven RDEB keratinocytes [15]. They further demonstrated that collagen VII expression may have a role in physical interaction with laminin-5 in the extracellular space, facilitating tumor invasion. However, more recently, this theory has been challenged by Pourreyron and colleagues, as they demonstrated that two out of eight RDEB-GS patient without detectable expression of collagen VII developed SCC [16]. The two RDEB-SCC patients had compound heterozygous nonsense mutations within the NC1 domain of collagen VII.

PREVENTION

As SCC in RDEB occurs frequently in a highly aggressive manner, regular detailed full body skin checks are vital for early detection and effective management. A few hospitals offer home visits by registered nurse to take photos, which are then assessed by medical professionals. This method may be more favored by RDEB patients as it is more convenient and they feel more comfortable at their homes. However, this method has disadvantages of being highly dependent on the quality of photos and has the potential to miss suspicious lesions, which may be more obvious through direct visualization by medical professionals [17].

The key to successful prevention of SCC is to have a high index of suspicion and to carefully inspect all areas of the body. The youngest age at which SCC has been reported in RDEB is 6 years [4]. In general, first SCC onset is in mid-adolescence or early twenties, and EB experts recommend a full skin check with all dressings removed to be performed every 3 months starting from at least age 12. Some patients are hesitant to undergo full skin checks because they feel embarrassed to have all their clothes and dressings removed, as well as having a fear of painful biopsies when suspicious areas are detected [17]. It is also a time-consuming process. Hence, it is important to have a warm room with a bathing facility prepared to ensure the patient's privacy and comfort.

Digital photographs need to be taken each visit for objective wound comparison with previous or upcoming visits. Our group has found that having the photos from each body area taken at the previous 3 months visit printed out and having them to hold directly next to the patient, as with mole checks, is the best way to compare the wounds, since some SCCs in RDEB often do not look like nodules and this is the best way to tell if a particular ulcer is lasting more than 3 months. This was how we realized that the wounds in our patients were healing and moving as their normal behavior pattern. Figure 1a-c show wound migration during skin checks every 3 months. If there is a suspicion of a premalignant or malignant lesion, such as a persistently painful lesion, one that is growing or an ulcer that has not healed in 3 months, it must be biopsied, ideally during the visit or as soon as possible. It is also important to encourage the patient and his/her family members to report on areas with persisting pain and poor healing. Assessments may be difficult as the appearance of a malignancy may be similar to that of a typical chronic ulceration. Therefore, biopsy should be performed with a low threshold [7]. In general, ulcerated areas persisting for more than 3 months without healing, painful areas, and hyperkeratotic nodules or plaques need to be biopsied as shown in Figure 2 [17]. Although rare, some cases of extracutaneous SCC such as SCC of the hard palate and oesophageal SCC have been reported in RDEB [18][19]. Lymph nodes need to be examined for detection of lymphatic spread, which will warrant a fine needle aspiration or lymph node excision biopsy [7]. Oral cavity and lymph node examination needs to be included for completion of a full skin check up. In Australia the new government-funded dressing scheme for EB allows the treating EB specialist to require reviews at certain frequencies, so patients with RDEB who do not attend for these essential reviews, do not get government-funded dressings. This encourages compliance with prevention and early detection strategies; we have experienced RDEB patients who previously received the dressings with no review of their skin on a regular basis developing skin cancers which were very advanced on presentation.

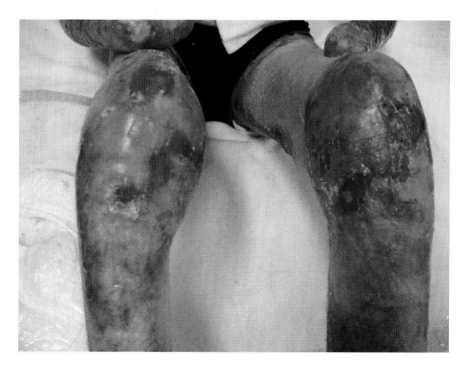

Figure 1a. Wound migration during a skin check (0 months).

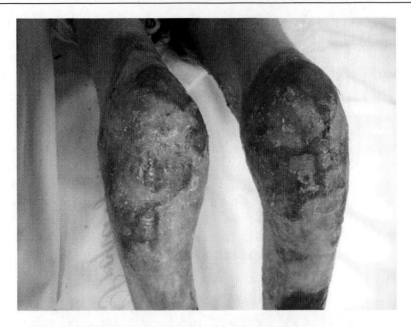

Figure 1b. Wound migration during a skin check (3 months).

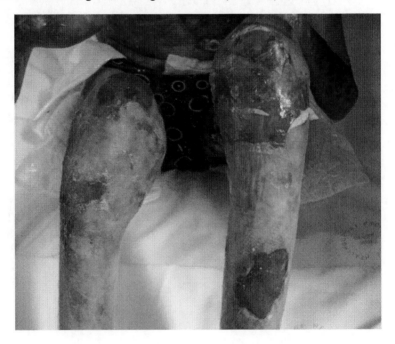

Figure 1c. Wound migration during a skin check (6 months).

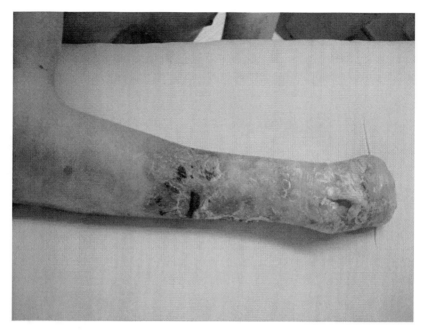

Figure 2. The hand of a patient with RDEB showing suspicious hyperkeratotic nodules and plaques that need to be biopsied.

A phase 1 trial of systemic isotretinoin demonstrated that RDEB patients have tolerated up to a dosage of 0.5mg/kg/d of isotretinoin, which may be used as a chemoprevention [20]. Common side effects from the use of isotretinoin include increased skin dryness and skin fragility. Low doses of neotigason were also tolerated well in a different group of RDEB patients [17].

TREATMENT

Once the diagnosis of SCC has been established through clinical history, physical examination, and skin biopsy, appropriate staging investigations should be performed using ultrasound, computerized tomography (CT) scans, magnetic resonance imaging (MRI), and positron emission tomography (PET) [17]. Prompt multidisciplinary team review involving the dermatologist, a plastic surgeon and a radiation oncologist who are familiar with EB should be instituted. Once local invasion has been detected, further imaging of the chest, abdomen, and pelvis is warranted. An MRI is particularly useful in determining tendon involvement and presence of extensive local spread. A

PET scan is especially useful for detection of haematogenous and lymphatic metastases that are difficult to visualize on a CT scan or MRI. Sentinel lymph node biopsies can be a useful tool in staging and determining prognosis while limiting morbidity during the process [21][22].

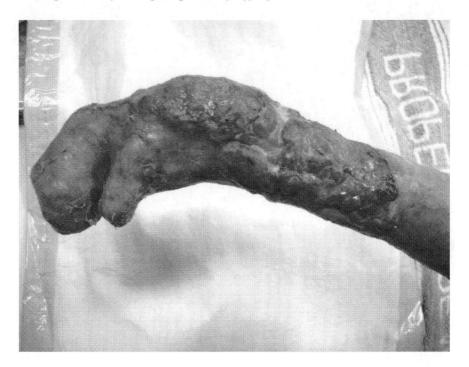

Figure 3a. A patient with an SCC on her hand.

Primary SCC without metastases in RDEB and JEB patients are treated by surgical means with full thickness excision with wide margins [17]. For SCC located in the extremities, local wide excision should be recommended under nerve blocks and spinal anaesthesia [23]. However, any presence of blisters and erosions on the back contraindicates spinal anaesthesia as this may lead to widespread bacterial infection. In such patients, general anaesthesia is warranted but oral intubation should be discouraged due to fragile mucosa. Therefore, a facial or laryngeal mask is preferred. Determining the extent of local spread is especially important in limb-sparing surgical options such as local wide excision. In the presence of tumor invasion of adjacent tendons or soft tissue without any evidence of distant metastases, amputation is warranted to prevent recurrence. Figures 3a-c show a patient with an SCC on her hand, axillary recurrence, and amputation. However, there is a lack of any supporting evidence for such circumstances and it is often difficult to detect any small distant metastasis. Reconstruction after tumor resection can be successfully performed with split-thickness skin grafts in EB patients, however, severe RDEB patient often lack normal suitable skin for grafting and require prolonged time for re-epithelialization after split-thickness harvest [23]. Thus, most surgeons recommend local skin flaps for reconstruction in RDEB patients.

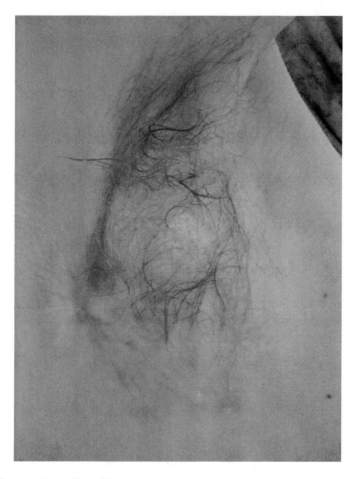

Figure 3b. A patient with axillary recurrence.

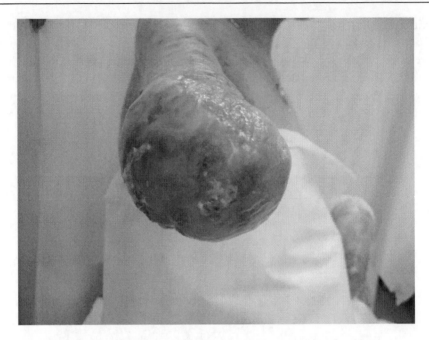

Figure 3c. A patient who had amputation of her arm due to an invasive SCC.

Chemotherapy and/or radiotherapy may be offered with surgical intervention. Currently, there is a lack of evidence in the literature on the role of adjuvant or neoadjuvant treatment regimens for SCC in EB. According to the NEBR in United States, only 5.7% and 17% of RDEB patients with metastatic SCC received chemotherapy and radiotherapy respectively [1]. Nevertheless, radiotherapy is valuable in reducing tumor size for surgery. With widespread metastatic disease, treatment is mostly palliative. Limb-sparing surgery to control local disease is recommended to improve the patient's quality of life. There is no consensus on drug choice for chemotherapy, dosage and duration. Furthermore radiotherapy is often delayed or discouraged by radiation oncologists due to the fear of skin toxicity. Palliative radiation may be valuable for improving quality of life in those with a symptomatic tumor mass.

Cetuximab, a monoclonal antibody against the epidermal growth factor receptor (EGFR), is currently used for advanced head and neck squamous cell cancers, colorectal cancers and some lung cancers of squamous cell origin. Overexpression of EGFR in tumor cells led to uncontrolled tumor growth and cetuximab has shown much benefit in these cancers. There have been cases of cetuximab use in RDEB-related SCC with full regression of the tumor in patients with metastatic disease [24][25]. Thus, cetuximab may be used as a first line treatment of unresectable or metastatic disease with radiotherapy or chemotherapy. Figure 4 shows a patient's stump with necrosis after radiotherapy and cetuximab.

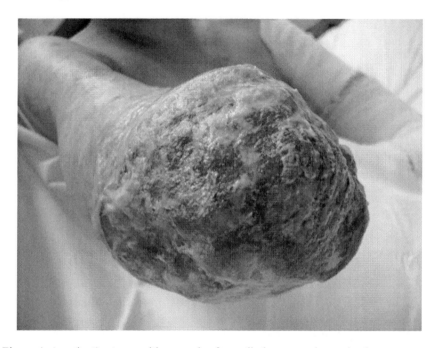

Figure 4. A patient's stump with necrosis after radiotherapy and cetuximab.

SUMMARY

SCC in the setting of EB is primarily related to RDEB and less often, JEB. It is not related to UV exposure but rather chronic repetitive wounds. The exact mechanism is to be determined but a number of factors have been discovered which may serve as therapeutic targets. Prevention from trauma, to reduce blistering, and early detection by comprehensive examination using digital photography every 3 months, ideally by the same experts, may allow for curative early excision. Some additional therapies, such as tyrosine kinase inhibitors, and retinoids have shown promising results. EB patients can tolerate radiotherapy as an adjunct to surgery. Chemotherapy is a very last resort, due to the risk of sepsis from chronically colonized skin. Research into the cause and better treatments for SCC, the major life threatening complication of RDEB, is one of the highest priorities in EB at present.

REFERENCES

[1]   Fine JD, Johnson LB, Weiner M et al. Epidermolysis bullosa and the risk of life-threatening cancers: The National EB Registry experience, 1986-2006. *Journal of the American Academy of Dermatology.* 60(2):203-11, 2009 Feb.

[2]   Ayman T, Yerebakan O, Ciftcioglu MA et al. A 13-year-old girl with recessive dystrophic epidermolysis bullosa presenting with squamous cell carcinoma. *Pediatric Dermatology.* 19(5):436-8, 2002 Sep-Oct.

[3]   Kawasaki H, Sawamura D, Iwao F et al. Squamous cell carcinoma developing in a 12-year-old boy with nonHallopeau-Siemens recessive dystrophic epidermolysis bullosa. *British Journal of Dermatology.* 148(5):1047-50, 2003 May.

[4]   Shivaswamy KN, Sumathy TK, Shyamprasad AL et al. Squamous cell carcinoma complicating epidermolysis bullosa in a 6-year-old girl. International *Journal of Dermatology.* 48(7):731-3, 2009 Jul.

[5]   McGrath JA, Schofield OMV, Mayou BJ et al. Epidermolysis bullosa complicated by squamous cell carcinoma: report of 10 cases. *Journal of Cutaneous Pathology.* 19(2):116-23, 1992 Apr.

[6]   Reed WB, College J, Francis MJO et al. Epidermolysis bullosa dystrophica with epidermal neoplasms *Archives of Dermatology.* 110(6):894-902, 1974 Dec.

[7]   Mallipeddi R. Epidermolysis bullosa and cancer. *Clinical and Experimental Dermatology.* 27: 616-23, 2002.

[8]   Goldberg GI, Eisen AZ & Bauer EA. Tissue stress and tumor promotion. *Archives of Dermatology.* 124(5):737-42, 1988 May.

[9]   Smoller BA, McNutt NS, Carter DM et al. Recessive dystrophic epidermolysis bullosa skin displays a chronic growth-activated immunophenotype. Implications for carcinogenesis. *Archives of Dermatology.* 126(1):78-83, 1990 Jan.

[10] Tyring SK, Chopra V, Johnson L et al. Natural killer cell activity is reduced in patients with severe forms of inherited epidermolysis bullosa. *Archives of Dermatology.* 125(6):797-800, 1989 Jun.

[11] Chopra V, Tyring SK, Johnson L et al. Patients with severe forms of inherited epidermolysis bullosa exhibit decreased lymphokine and monokine production. *Journal of Clinical Immunology.* 10(6):321-9, 1990 Nov.

[12] Arbiser JL, Fine JD, Murrell D et al. Basic fibroblast growth factor: a missing link between collagen VII, increased collagenase, and squamous cell carcinoma in recessive dystrophic epidermolysis bullosa. *Molecular Medicine.* 4(3):191-5, 1998 March.

[13] D'Armiento J, SiColandrea T, Dalal SS et al. Collagenase expression in transgenic mouse skin causes hyperkeratosis and acanthosis and increases susceptibility to tumorigenesis. *Molecular and Cellular Biology.* 15(10):5732-9, 1995 Oct.

[14] Kivisaari AK, Kallajoki M, Mirtti T et al. Transformation-specific matrix metalloproteinases (MMP)-7 and MMP-13 are expressed by tumour cells in epidermolysis bullosa-associated squamous cell carcinomas. *British Journal of Dermatology.* 158(4):778-85, 2008 Apr.

[15] Ortiz-Urda S, Garcia J, Green CL et al. Type VII collagen is required for ras-driven human epidermal tumorigenesis. *Science.* 307(5716):1773-6, 2005 Mar.

[16] Pourreyron C, Cox G, Mao X et al. Patients with recessive dystrophic epidermolysis bullosa develop squamous-cell carcinoma regardless of type VII collagen expression. *Journal of Investigative Dermatology.* 127(10):2438-44, 2007 Oct.

[17] Venugopal SS & Murrell DF. Treatment of skin cancers in epidermolysis bullosa. *Dermatologic Clinics.* 28(2):283-7, 2010 Apr.

[18] Martinez L, Goodman P, Crow WN. Squamous cell carcinoma of the maxillary sinus and plaque in epidermolysis bullosa: CT demonstration. *Journal of Computer Assisted Tomography.* 16(2): 317-9, 1992.

[19] Ray A, Bhattacharya S, Kumar A et al. Rare occurrence of carcinoma oesophagus in a case of epidermolysis bullosa. *Indian Journal of Cancer.* 46(1): 72-3, 2009 Jan-Mar, 2009.

[20] Fine JD, Johnson LB, Weiner M et al. Chemoprevention of squamous cell carcinoma in recessive dystrophic epidermolysis bullosa: results of a phase 1 trial of systemic isotretinoin. *Journal of the American Academy of Dermatology.* 50(4):563-71, 2004 Apr. 2004.

[21] Rokunohe A, Nakano H, Aizu T et al. Significance of sentinel node biopsy in the management of squamous cell carcinoma arising from recessive dystrophic epidermolysis bullosa. *Journal of Dermatology.* 35(6):336-40, 2008 Jun.

[22] Perez-Naranjo L, Herrera-Saval A, Garcia-Bravo B et al. Sentinel lymph node biopsy in recessive dystrophic epidermolysis bullosa and squamous cell carcinoma. *Archives of Dermatology*. 141(1):110-1, 2005 Jan.

[23] Yamada M, Hatta N, Sogo K et al. Management of squamous cell carcinoma in a patient with recessive-type epidermolysis bullosa dystrophica. *Dermatologic Surgery*. 30(11):1424-9, 2004 Nov.

[24] Arnold AW, Bruckner-Tuderman L, Zuger C et al. Cetuximab therapy of metastasizing cutaneous squamous cell carcinoma in a patient with severe recessive dystrophic epidermolysis bullosa. *Dermatology*. 219(1):80-3, 2009 May.

[25] Maubec E, Petrow P, Duvillard P et al. Cetuximab as first-line monotherapy in patients with unresectable squamous cell carcinoma of the skin: preliminary results of a phase II multicenter study. *Journal of Clinical Oncology*. 26(May 20 suppl); abstr 9042, 2008 May

In: Squamous Cell Carcinoma
Editor: Daniel V. Mortensen

ISBN: 978-1-61209-929-3
© 2012 Nova Science Publishers, Inc.

Chapter 6

DYNAMIC ALTERATION OF NUCLEOLIN AND AgNOR PROTEINS IN ORAL CANCER APOPTOTIC CELLS BY ULTRAVIOLET RAYS IRRADIATION

Shinji Kito[1], Shunji Shiiba[2], Masafumi Oda[1],
Tatsurou Tanaka[1], Yuji Seta[3], Nao Wakasugi-Sato[1],
Shinobu Matsumoto-Takeda[1], Izumi Yoshioka[4], and
Yasuhiro Morimoto[*1, 5,]

[1] Department of Oral Diagnostic Science, Kyushu Dental College,
Kitakyushu, Japan
[2] Department of Control of Physical Functions,
Kyushu Dental College, Kitakyushu, Japan
[3] Department of Bioscience, Kyushu Dental College, Kitakyushu, Japan
[4] Department of Sensory and Motor Organs, Faculty of Medicine,
Miyazaki University, Miyazaki, Japan
[5] Center for Oral Biological Research, Kyushu Dental College,
Kitakyushu, Japan

---

* Send all correspondence to: Yasuhiro Morimoto DDS PhD, Division of Diagnostic Radiology, Department of Oral Diagnostic Science, Kyushu Dental College, 2-6-1 Manazuru, Kokurakita-ku, Kitakyushu 803-8580, JAPAN, TEL: 81-93-285-3094, FAX: 81-93-285-3094,　　　　　　　　E-mail:　　　　　　　　Rad-Mori@Kyu-Dent.Ac.Jp

ABSTRACT

The behavior of nucleolin and AgNOR proteins in ultraviolet (UV) irradiation-induced apoptosis of oral cancer cells was investigated. In addition, the alteration of nucleolin and AgNORs proteins in apoptotic oral cancer cells induced by okadaic acid and anti-cancer drugs in our previous studies was reviewed. Dynamic alterations of nucleolin and AgNORs proteins in UV irradiation-induced apoptotic HSG cells were visualized using Western blot analysis and histocytochemistry methods. It was found that the 110-kDa forms of nucleolin and AgNOR proteins decreased in quantity, while the 80- and 95-kDa forms appeared during apoptosis caused by UV exposure in apoptotic HSG cells. Nucleolin disappeared or diffusely spread out into the nucleus in the apoptotic body of oral cancer cells. Based on this and previous reports, alteration of nucleolin, an AgNOR-associated protein, is associated with the induction of DNA fragmentation in the final active phase of apoptosis in oral cancer cells.

Keywords: oral cancer cells; apoptosis; ultra-violet rays; anti-cancer drugs

INTRODUCTION

Molecular defects in apoptotic pathways are thought to often contribute to the abnormal expansion of malignant cells and to their resistance to chemotherapy and radiotherapy [1, 2]. Therefore, a comprehensive knowledge of the mechanisms controlling the induction of apoptosis and the subsequent cellular disintegration could result in improved methods for the treatment of cancer and a better prognosis [1, 2].

Apoptosis is a form of self-regulated cell death that occurs during development, immune regulation, and normal cell turnover; it may also be induced by pharmacological agents [1-3]. The characteristic morphological changes of apoptosis include cytoplasmic shrinkage, plasma membrane blebbing, chromatin condensation, and formation of apoptotic bodies containing well-preserved organelles [1-3]. The most distinctive morphological features of apoptosis are cell rounding, cell shrinking, and condensation of the nucleus as in mitosis [3]. From such condensation, it may be inferred that the alteration of nuclear proteins is also related to apoptosis. It has been reported that the morphological changes that occur during apoptosis may be induced by the alteration of various nuclear matrix proteins [2-9], including lamin B [6], nuclear mitotic apparatus protein (NuMA) [7], argyrophilic nucleolar organizer region (AgNOR) proteins [8], and nucleolin [2, 8, 9].

In Particular, Nucleolin And Agnor Proteins Seem To Play Important Roles In Cell Growth, Proliferation, And Apoptosis [2]. In Our Previous Studies, We Found That Alteration Of Nucleolin And Agnor Proteins Was Induced By A Protein Phosphatase Inhibitor In Cultured Cells [8, 9]. In Addition, We Demonstrated That The Characteristic Alterations Of Nucleolin And Agnor Proteins Occurred In Anti-Cancer Drug-Induced Apoptotic Oral Cancer Cells [10]. Our Previous Studies Suggest That Alterations Of Nucleolin And Agnor Proteins Are Associated With The Induction Of DNA Fragmentation And The Final Active Phase Of Apoptosis Induced By Anti-Cancer Drugs In Oral Cancer Cells [8-10]. In The Present Article, We Review The Alterations Of Nucleolin And Agnor Proteins In Our Previous Studies And New Data Related To Ultraviolet (UV)-Induced Apoptotic Oral Cancer Cells.

INDUCTION OF APOPTOSIS BY VARIOUS STIMULATORS INCLUDING UV IRRADIATION IN ORAL CELLS

UV irradiation and anti-cancer drugs may be thought to directly attack the double and single strands of DNA and thus induce cytotoxicity and cellular apoptosis [3]. At the same time, unusual phosphorylation and dephosphorylation may be induced by UV irradiation. Certainly, UV irradiation also significantly increased the incidence of apoptosis in human submandibular gland ductal cell line (HSG) cells in an exposure volume-dependent manner, as demonstrated by DNA ladder formation, as has also been seen in apoptosis induced by okadaic acid and anti-cancer drugs. [8-10] The use of okadaic acid (OA) has led to the understanding that phosphorylation and dephosphorylation status is related to cell proliferation and differentiation in mammalian cells. Anti-cancer drugs may directly attack the double and single strands of DNA and thus induce cytotoxicity and cellular apoptosis. [10] Figure 1 shows that UV irradiation induces apoptosis in HSG cells in an exposure volume-dependent manner. In UV-irradiated cells, a DNA fragmentation pattern forming a ladder with multiples of 185-200 bp was observed (Fig. 1A). Okadaic acid [8, 9, 11, 12] and anti-cancer drugs [10] also induced apoptosis in oral cancers cells in an exposure time-dependent manner. In anti-cancer drug-treated HSG cells, a DNA fragmentation pattern forming a ladder with multiples of 185-200 bp was observed (Fig. 1B). [10] The stability of DNA double strand and protein phosphorylation/dephosphorylation may be a key mechanism in the regulation of apoptosis in various tissues. Therefore, we paid attention to two of the nuclear proteins, nucleolin and AgNOR proteins, and investigated the alterations of these proteins in apoptotic oral cancer cells by apoptosis stimulators including UV irradiation. [8-12]

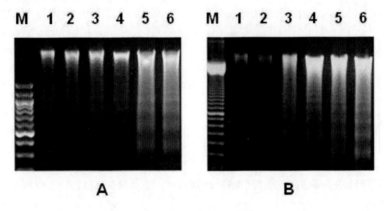

Figure 1. Effects of UV irradiation and anti-cancer drug administration on HSG cells. (A) DNA ladder formation. Subconfluent HSG cells were exposed to UV irradiation for various lengths of time. Lane M, standard DNA markers (bp); lane 1, unexposed control cells; lane 2, cells irradiated for 7 J/m^2; lane 3, 10 J/m^2; lane 4, 14 J/m^2; lane 5, 30 J/m^2, and lane 6, 60 J/m^2. (B) Effects of cisplatin on HSG cells. DNA ladder formation in HSG cells treated with cisplatin. Subconfluent HSG cells were exposed for 24 h with various concentrations. Lane 1, untreated control cells; lane 2, cells treated with 0.5 μM cisplatin; lane 3, 5 μM; lane 4, 25 μM; lane 5, 50 μM, and lane 6, 100 μM.

Nucleolin has many functions, including its role in mitosis and its ability to translocate within cells [2, 8, 9, 10,13-26]. This protein is associated with the dysfunctional processes of proliferation, cell cycle control, and apoptosis in neoplastic cells; in addition, elevated levels of nucleolin expression are generally related to malignancy [2, 13, 14].

ALTERATION OF NUCLEOLIN AND AGNOR PROTEINS IN ORAL CELL APOPTOSIS INDUCED BY STIMULATORS, INCLUDING UV IRRADIATION

We investigated the alterations of nucleolin and AgNOR proteins during apoptosis induced by UV irradiation in oral cancer cells using Western blot analysis and histocytochemistry methods, as we did with okaic acid and anticancer drugs [8-10] (Figures 2 and 3). The 110-kDa form of nucleolin decreased in quantity, while the 80- and 95-kDa forms appeared during apoptosis in cultured oral cancer cells (Figures 2 and 3). In addition, on histocytochemical analysis, nucleolin and AgNOR proteins disappeared or diffusely spread out into the nucleus in the apoptotic bodies of oral cancer cells (Figures 4 and 5). [8-10]

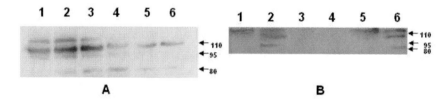

Figure 2. Identification of nucleolin in HSG cells (A) and HSG cells (B) using Western blot analysis. (A) Subconfluent cells were exposed to various volumes of UV irradiation for various lengths of time, and cellular proteins were prepared. Lane 1, unexposed control cells; lane 2, cells irradiated for 7 J/m^2; lane 3, 10 J/m^2; lane 4, 14 J/m^2; lane 5, 30 J/m^2, and lane 6, 60 J/m^2. (B) Subconfluent HSG cells were exposed to UV irradiation for 14 J/m^2 and the cellular proteins were prepared. Whole cell lysates (1 and 2), cytosolic fractions (3 and 4), and nuclear fractions (5 and 6) were prepared from unexposed cells (1, 3, and 5) or UV irradiation-induced apoptotic cells (2, 4, and 6). The molecular weight is indicated along the right side in kDa.

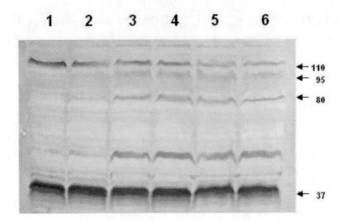

Figure 3. Identification of AgNOR proteins in HSG cells using modified Western blot analysis. Subconfluent HSG cells were exposed to various volumes of UV. The molecular weight is indicated along the right side in kDa. Lane 1, unexposed control cells; lane 2, cells irradiated for 7 J/m^2; lane 3, 10 J/m^2; lane 4, 14 J/m^2; lane 5, 30 J/m^2, and lane 6, 60 J/m^2.

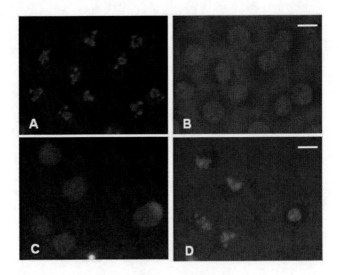

Figure 4. Identification of nucleolin in HSG cells. Apoptosis was induced by UV irradiation by 14 J/m^2. The staining methods are described in the Materials and Methods section. Unexposed control cells were stained with anti-nucleolin antibody (A) or Hoechst 33342 (B). The UV-irradiated cells were stained with anti-nucleolin antibody (C) or Hoechst 33342 (D). The bar represents 10 μm.

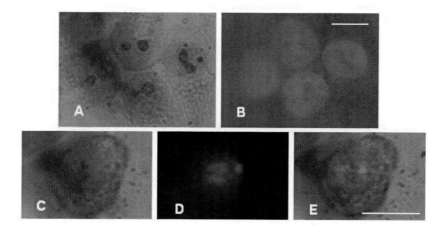

Figure 5. Cytochemical identification of AgNORs in apoptotic HSG cells. Apoptosis was induced by UV irradiation at 14 J/m^2. The staining method is described in the Materials and Methods section. Untreated control cells were stained with AgNO$_3$ (A) and Hoechst 33342 (B). Apoptotic cells also were stained with AgNO$_3$ (C) and Hoechst 33342 (D). Figure 5E is a superimposition of Figures 5C and 5D. The bar represents 10 μm.

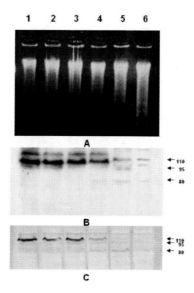

Figure 6. The time course of DNA fragmentation (A) and alteration of nucleolin (B) and AgNOR proteins (C) in nuclei from HSG cells treated with cytosolic extracts from apoptotic HSG cells. Intact nuclei were incubated with the cytosolic fraction of control HSG cells or treated for 14 h with 50 μM cisplatin. The DNA was extracted and

electrophoresed through an agarose gel, yielding a ladder pattern (A). Each 20-μl reaction mixture described in the Material and Methods section underwent Western blot analysis for nucleolin (B) or modified Western blot analysis for AgNOR proteins (C). The molecular weight is indicated along the right side in kDa. Lane 1, untreated control cells; lane 2, cells treated for 0 minute; lane 3, 15 minutes; lane 4, 30 minutes; lane 5, 60 minutes, and lane 6, 120 minutes.

Several studies have examined the role of nucleolin in cell death. Martelli et al. reported a redistribution of nucleolin (associated with the fragmentation of nuclei) in apoptotic cells but not necrotic cells and reported that nucleolin was not degraded during apoptosis [23-25]. Mi et al. also suggested that nucleolin was not degraded during apoptosis [2]. Conversely, Brockstedt et al. used two-dimensional electrophoresis to identify nucleolin as a protein that was cleaved in a Burkitt's lymphoma cell line [26]. In our previous studies using okadaic acid and anti-cancer drugs, cleavage of nucleolin was observed during apoptosis in various kinds of cultured cells and in a cell-free apoptotic system (Figures 6) [8-10]. Mi et al. suggested that the cause of the contradictory findings regarding apoptosis-induced cleavage of nucleolin might be cell death occurring via different mechanisms [2]. However, using UV irradiation, the 110-kDa form of nucleolin decreased in quantity, while the 80- and 95-kDa forms appeared during apoptosis in cultured oral cancer cells (Figures 2 and 3).

CHARACTERISTICS OF ALTERNATIVE NUCLEOLIN AND AGNOR PROTEINS WITH UV IRRADIATION-INDUCED APOPTOSIS

Further study is needed focusing on the appearance of the 80- and 95-kDa forms of nucleolin in UV irradiation-induced apoptotic oral cancer cells. Whether the 95-kDa protein is a cleaved form or a dephosphorylated form of nucleolin is not presently clear. The amount of the 95-kDa protein decreased in MG 63 cells treated with okadaic acid, a protein phosphatase inhibitor [9]. The protein phosphatase type 1 δ isoform is reportedly associated with nucleolin and might dephosphorylate it [27]. These findings suggest that nucleolin could be partially dephosphorylated into a 95-kDa protein in the initial phase of apoptosis [9, 27]. The amounts of the 95-kDa protein increased in oral cancer cells with UV irradiation.

We speculated that, in UV irradiation-induced apoptotic cells, in the dynamic alteration of nucleolin, initially some 110-kDa nucleolins might be partially dephosphorylated into 95-kDa proteins, while other 110-kDa nucleolins might be cleaved into 80-kDa proteins. However, as another possibility, 95-kDa nucleolins might be partially proteolyzed into the 80-kDa protein during preparation.

Therefore, the alteration of nucleolin in apoptosis might be an indicator of universal cell change. The alterations of nucleolin and AgNOR proteins may be useful markers for the presence of apoptosis. Because the detection method of AgNOR proteins is much easier, the alteration of AgNOR proteins may be more popular as a clinical and experimental indicator for apoptotic cells. Of course, the cause of the contradictory results might be the characteristics of the respective cells; further study is necessary to clarify the cause.

RELATIONSHIP BETWEEN DNA LADDER FORMATION AND THE ALTERATIONS OF NUCLEOLIN AND AGNOR PROTEINS

A relationship was found between the time of detectable DNA ladder formation and the alteration of nucleolin from 110-kDa to 80-kDa in the apoptotic cells and in the cell-free apoptotic system (Figure 6) [8-10]. When normal nuclei were irradiated and then directly mixed with normal cytoplasm in an apoptotic cell-free system, DNA ladder formation and cleavage of nucleolin from 110-kDa into 80-kDa proteins were still detectable. These findings directly proved that the cleavage of nucleolin might be related to apoptosis. Nucleolin may play an important role in the executive phase of apoptosis. Activation of at least one nuclease through unknown mechanisms may cleave the nucleolin, which in turn activates at least one endonuclease, resulting in DNA ladder formation. However, the precise role of nucleolin in apoptosis has not yet been elucidated.

The nucleolin changes in UV irradiation-induced apoptosis and in anti-cancer drug-induced apoptosis [11] are contradictory to the ones in protein phosphatase inhibitor-induced apoptosis. One possible explanation for this contradiction may be the difference in the mechanisms of cell injury between UV irradiation and anti-cancer drugs [3, 10] and protein phosphatase inhibitors [8, 9, 11, 12]. The protein phosphatase inhibitor okadaic acid is thought to act in the cytoplasm and/or on the proteins of the cell surface through the Fas/Fas ligand system to induce apoptosis [12]. However, UV irradiation and anti-cancer drugs are thought to directly attack the double and single strands of DNA and thus induce cytotoxicity and apoptosis in the cells [3, 10].

Regarding the cleavage of 110-kDa nucleolin into 95-, 80-, and 75-kDa forms, incubation of nucleolin with granzyme A reportedly generates a discrete proteolytic cleavage product of 88-kDa in vitro [28]. An 80-kDa nucleolin may be a proteolytic fragment form of a 110-kDa nucleolin cleaved by novel proteases. The proteases involved may be similar to granzyme A [29]. Because it has been reported that the apoptosis-inducing granzyme A and interleukin-1 β converting enzyme (ICE) share at least one substrate, pre-interleukin (pI)L-1 [29], the changes in nucleolin might be induced by ICE. Direct investigation of nucleolin structure during apoptosis may be facilitated by purification of nucleolin and immunoblotting with anti-nucleolin antibodies. Identification of any proteases involved in the cleavage of nucleolin is needed to further understand the executive phase of apoptosis. Regulation of nucleolin cleavage might regulate the executive phase of apoptosis including UV irradiation-, anti-cancer drug-, and okadaic acid-induced cytotoxicity. Further study is also needed to clarify how the fragments of nucleolin are transported from the nucleus to the cytoplasm during apoptosis.

ACKNOWLEDGMENTS

This study was supported in part by grants-in-aid for scientific research from the Ministry of Education, Science, Sports and Culture of Japan, from the President of Kyushu Dental College, and from Kitakyushu City to YM.

REFERENCES

[1]   Kerr JFR, Winterford CM, Harmon BV. Apoptosis: Its significance in cancer and cancer therapy. *Cancer* 1994; 73: 2013-26.
[2]   Mi Y, Thomas SD, Xu X, Casson LK, Miller DM, Bates PJ. Apoptosis in leukemia cells is accompanied by alterations in the levels and localization of nucleolin. J Biol Chem 2003; 278: 8572-9.

[3]   Steller H. Mechanisms and genes of cellular suicide. *Science* 1995; 267: 1445-9.

[4]   Casciola-Rosen LA, Miller DK, Anhalt GJ, Rosen A. Specific cleavage of 70-kDa protein component of the U1 small nuclear ribonucleoprotein is a characteristic biochemical feature of apoptotic cell death. *J Biol Chem* 1994; 269: 30757-60.

[5]   Brockstedt E, Richers A, Kostka S, Laubersheimer A, Dorken B, Wittmann-Liebold B, Bommert K, Otto A. Identification of apoptosis-associated proteins in a human Burkitt lymphoma cell line. Cleavage of heterogeneous nuclear ribonucleoprotein A1 by caspase 3. *J Biol Chem* 1998; 273: 28057-64.

[6]   Neamati N, Fernandez A, Wright S, Kiefer J, McConkey DJ. Degradation of lamin B1 precedes oligonucleosomal DNA fragmentation in apoptotic thymocytes and isolated thymocyte nuclei. *J Immunol* 1995; 154: 3788-95.

[7]   Gueth-Hallonet C, Weber K, Osborn M. Cleavage of the nuclear matrix protein NuMA during apoptosis. *Exp Cell Res* 1995; 233: 21-4.

[8]   Morimoto Y, Kito S, Ohba T, Morimoto H, Okamura H and Haneji T. Alteration of argyrophilic nucleolar organizer region associated (Ag-NOR) proteins in apoptosis-induced human salivary gland cells and human oral squamous carcinoma cells. *J Oral Pathol Med* 2001; 30: 193-9.

[9]   Kito S, Shimizu K, Okamura H, Yoshida K, Morimoto H, Fujita M, Morimoto Y, Ohba T, and Haneji T. Cleavage of nucleolin and argyrophilic nucleolar organizer region associated proteins in apoptosis-induced cells. *Biochem Biophys Res Commun* 2003; 300: 950-6.

[10]   Kito S, Morimoto Y, Tanaka T, Haneji T, Ohba T: Cleavage of nucleolin and AgNOR proteins during apoptosis induced by anti-cancer drugs in human salivary gland cells. *J Oral Pathol Med* 2005; 34: 478-85.

[11]   Morimoto Y, Ohba T, Kobayashi S, Haneji T. The protein phosphatase inhibitors okadaic acid and calyculin A induce apoptosis in human osteoblastic cells. *Exp Cell Res* 1997; 230: 181-6.

[12]   Morimoto Y, Morimoto H, Okamura H, Nomiyama K, Nakamuta N, Kobayashi S, Kito S, Ohba T, and Haneji T. Okadaic acid up-regulates expression of Fas antigen and Fas ligand in human submandibular gland ductal cell line HSG cells. *Arch Oral Biol* 2000; 45: 657-66.

[13]   Walker RA. The histopathological evaluation of nucleolar organizer region proteins. *Histopathology* 1988; 12: 221-3.

134   Shinji Kito, Shunji Shiiba, Masafumi Oda et al.

[14] Underwood JC, Giri DD. Nucleolar organizer regions as diagnostic discriminants for malignancy. *J Pathol* 1988; 155: 95-6.

[15] Ochs RL, Busch H. Further evidence that phosphoprotein C23 (110 kD/pI 5.1) is the nucleolar silver staining protein. *Exp Cell Res* 1984; 152: 260-5.

[16] Borer RA, Lehner CF, Eppenberger HM, Nigg EA. Major nucleolar proteins shuttle between nucleus and cytoplasm. *Cell* 1989; 56: 379-90.

[17] Ochs R, Lischwe M, O'Leary P, Busch H. Localization of nucleolar phosphoproteins B23 and C23 during mitosis. *Exp Cell Res* 1983; 146: 139-49.

[18] Morimoto H, Okamura H, Haneji T. Interaction of protein phosphatase 1δ with nucleolin in human osteoblastic cells. *J Histochem Cytochem* 2002; 50: 1187-93.

[19] Chen CM, Chiang SY, Yeh NH. Increased stability of nucleolin in proliferating cells by inhibition of its self-cleaving activity. *J Biol Chem* 1991; 266: 7754-8.

[20] Mateli MS, Bleier KJ, Mcinerney TN. Granzyme A binding to target cells proteins. Granzyme A binds to and cleaves nucleolin in vitro. *J Biol Chem* 1991; 266: 14703-8.

[21] Pasternack MS, Bleier KJ, McInerney TN. Granzyme A binding to target cell proteins. Granzyme A binds to and cleaves nucleolin in vitro. *J Biol Chem* 1991; 266: 14703-8.

[22] Gilchrist JSC, Abrenica B, DiMario PJ, Czubryt MP, Pierce GN. Nucleolin is a calcium-binding protein. *J Cell Biochem* 2002; 85: 268-78.

[23] Martelli AM, Robuffo I, Bortul R, Ochs RL, Luchetti, F, Cocco L, Zweyer M, Bareggi R, Falcieri E. *J Cell Biochem* 2000; 78, 264-77.

[24] Bortul R, Zweyer M, Billi AM, Tabellini G, Ochs RL, Bareggi R, Cocco L, Martelli AM. *J Cell Biochem* 2001; 81, 19-31.

[25] Martelli AM, Zweyer M, Ochs RL, Tazzari PL, Tabellini G, Narducci P, Bortul R. *J Cell Biochem* 2000; 82, 634-46.

[26] Brockstedt E, Rickers A, Kostka S, Laubersheimer A, Dorken B, Wittmann-Liebold B, Bommert K, Otto A. *J Biol Chem* 1998; 273, 28057-64.

[27] Morimoto H, Okamura H, Haneji H. Interaction of protein phosphatases 1δ with nucleolin in human osteoblastic cells. *J Histochem Cytochem* 2002; 50: 1187-93.

[28] Paternack MS, Bleier KJ, McInerney TN. Granzyme A binding to target cell protein. Granzyme A binds to and cleaves nucleolin in vitro. *J Biol Chem* 1991; 266: 14703-8.

[29] Irmler M, Hertig S, MacDonald HR, et al. Granzyme A is an interleukin 1b-converting enzyme. *J Exp Med* 1995; 181: 1917-22.

In: Squamous Cell Carcinoma   ISBN: 978-1-61209-929-3
Editor: Daniel V. Mortensen   © 2012 Nova Science Publishers, Inc.

Chapter 7

SQUAMOUS CELL CARCINOMA OF TONGUE: LESS INVASIVE SURGICAL APPROACHES TO TONGUE CARCINOMAS

Masaaki Kodama[*,1], *Amit Khanal*[1,2], *Manabu Habu*[1],
Izumi Yoshioka[1,3], *Takeshi Nishikawa*[1],
Hiroki Tsurushima[1], *Yusuke Yanagida*[1], *Shinji Kito*[4],
Tatsurou Tanaka[4], *Yasuhiro Morimoto*[4] and
Kazuhiro Tominaga[1]

[1]Division of Maxillofacial Diagnostic and Surgical Science,
Department of Oral and Maxillofacial Surgery,
Kyushu Dental College, Kitakyushu, Japan
[2]Department of Oral and Maxillofacial Surgery,
B.P. Koirala Institute of Health Sciences, Dharan, Nepal
[3]Department of Oral and Maxillofacial Surgery, Faculty of Medicine,
Miyazaki University, Miyazaki, Japan
[4]Division of Diagnostic Radiology, Department of Oral Diagnostic
Science, Kyushu Dental College, Kitakyushu, Japan

---

* Send all correspondence to: Masaaki Kodama DDS PhD, Division of Maxillofacial Diagnostic
and Surgical Science, Department of Oral and Maxillofacial Surgery, Kyushu Dental
College, 2-6-1 Manazuru, Kokurakita-ku, Kitakyushu 803-8580, JAPAN, TEL: 81-93-582-
1131, FAX: 81-93-582-1286, E-mail: m-kodama@kyu-dent.ac.jp

ABSTRACT

Tongue is one of the most common sites of oral squamous cell carcinomas (SCC). A good treatment strategy should incorporate an optimal resection with adequate surgical clearance and minimal physical dysfunction. Surgical clearance depends on surgeon's experience as there are no available methods for intraoperative diagnosis. Ultrasonography (US) is increasingly being used in oral and maxillofacial regions for detection of soft tissue-related diseases like salivary gland tumors, regional lymph nodes, etc. US is non-invasive real time imaging technique especially suitable for detecting tumors of small dimensions that are not readable even by CT scan or MRI. At present, US is mainly used as a diagnostic aid. Early stage tongue carcinomas (T1-T2) are especially benefited by US. The use of US before resection of tongue carcinomas for approximate evaluation of tumor thickness is routinely carried out. This time, we propose a diagnostic and therapeutic intervention of US in tongue carcinomas to confirm the surgical clearance and safety margin intraoperatively using a new method.

Keywords: tongue, squamous cell carcinoma, ultrasonography, surgical clearance

Oral squamous cell carcinomas (SCC) with its aggressive nature especially when occurring in the tongue are likely to invade deeply due to its tendency to spread along muscle fibers, fascial planes and lymphatics. Tongue is divided into two anatomical parts, a mobile tongue (anterior two-thirds) and a fixed base tongue. Up to 75% of tongue SCC arises in anterior mobile part. The mobile tongue can be further subdivided into tip, lateral borders, dorsum, and ventral surface. Lateral border is the preponderant site for origin of carcinomas; accounting for three-quarters of it. The ventral surface is second in order of frequency with 12-15% of cases, followed by the dorsum (5-7%) and the tip (2-3%) [1]. The incidence of cervical metastasis in tongue SCC correlates with the T stage of primary tumor and appears to be significant even at early stages. The location of primary lesion on the tongue does not appear to be important with regard to metastasis to the lymph nodes (lateral border 27%, ventral tongue 24%, tip 22%, and dorsum 21%) [2]. However, extension of SCC to the oral floor is associated with an increased frequency of nodal metastasis.

Circumvallate papillae are anatomical landmarks that delineate the tongue into anterior mobile part and fixed posterior base. However, there are no barriers to prevent the carcinomas from spreading throughout the tongue. Further, there is an absence of barriers to cross-over into contralateral channels of the tongue's rich lymphatic drainage. Carcinomas arising at base-of-tongue are not readily visible for self-inspection, and hence often leading to discovery at a late stage. Besides, the aggressiveness of SCC of base-of-tongue can be appreciated by the fact that 50-75% of patients have clinically positive cervical lymph nodes at diagnosis and 20-30% either have, or will have contralateral and/or bilateral cervical nodal metastasis, almost three-quarters of carcinomas that have extended beyond base into the anterior tongue, pre-epiglottic space, pharyngeal walls, or mandible, about 20% will invade the larynx.

Many reports have shown that tumor thickness of tongue SCC is a very useful index. Spiro et al have shown that patients with tongue and oral floor carcinomas having 2mm or less thickness had a treatment failure rate of 1.9% compared with 45.6% for patients whose primary carcinomas were thicker than 2mm [3]. Rasgon et al showed a significant increase in the cervical lymph node metastasis with lesion more than 5mm thick as compared with those lesser than 5mm [4]. These data suggest that treatment failure and survival may be dependent more on tumor thickness than on clinical stages.

Despite significant advances in cancer therapy, i.e. advanced radiotherapy and chemotherapy, the survival rate of patients with tongue SCC has not changed over the last 3 decades. Although, surgical treatment of tongue SCC has not changed, surgery is still the most reliable therapy.

Generally, surgical margin of tongue SCC can be easily delineated on the mucosal surface with a certain safety margin. However, the deep surgical margin is usually determined by empirical fashion such as manipulation by surgeon's hands. Therefore, surgical resection depends on surgeon's experience, and hence may lead to a tendency to underestimate the tumor size and possible human error. A review of literature found close or involved margins in 20-50% of the studied resection cases [5]. So, several studies have shown that histological margins lesser than 5 mm from the tumor front have high local recurrence rates with diminished 5 years survival [6-8]. To achieve a minimum 5 mm of histological clearance after specimen shrinkage, resection margin of 10 mm during surgery is considered adequate to avoid any underestimation of the actual tumor size. Yet, another report advocated the clearance margin of 15-20mm to avoid any possibility of underestimation and technical error [9]. In our daily life, tongue has a lot of important roles like speech, taste, swallowing, etc. Although large safety clearance may lead to low recurrence, patient's QOL will remarkably decrease after surgery. Hence, enough safety clearance for its radicality as well as minimal invasion of normal tissues for functional aspect is very desirable. At present, there are no available methods to resect tongue carcinomas objectively and evaluate the clearance of surgical margin of the resected specimen intra-operatively.

Ultrasonography (US) is non-invasive real time imaging technique that is increasingly being used in oral and maxillofacial regions for diagnostic purposes and detection of soft tissue-related anomalies. There are many studies that have described the US features of metastatic cervical lymph nodes. At recent times, high resolution diagnostic intraoral US for accurate preoperative evaluation of tumor thickness of primary tongue carcinomas has become available. Shintani et al have shown a good correlation between the thickness determined by intraoral US measurement and histologically proven thickness [10]. They have also shown that US is superior to CT and MRI for measurement of any tumor thickness lesser than 5mm [11]. Yuen et al recently concluded that US had satisfactory accuracy for measurement of tumor thickness and its usefulness as an adjunctive technique for assisting pretreatment staging and prognostic evaluation of patients with oral tongue carcinomas [12]. Furthermore, Songra et al reported good reliability for intra-oral and intra-operative US imaging when objectively assessing tumor thickness and surgical margin clearance at the time of surgery [13]. Additional studies have similarly reported the exact assessment of tongue tumor thickness using intraoral US [14-18]. However, in most of these studies, tumor thickness of US images are not accurate owing to the fact of either lack of proper contacts between the US probe and the tumor surface or distortions in tumor's shape due to US probe's pressure. So, this time we propose a reliable method to confirm the surgical clearance and safety margin of tongue SCC using US intra-operatively.

The method in detail is described in our earlier published paper [19]. In brief, patient with tongue SCC was examined for tumor thickness initially with an SSD-1200CV US machine equipped with a 7.5 MHz sector probe (Aloka Ltd, Tokyo, Japan) under general anesthesia. Then elastic needle (20 gauge) with a metal core is introduced to indicate deep surgical margin clearance under continuous US monitoring (Fig. 1a). The tip of the needle was placed approximately 10 mm from the deepest portion of the tumor invasion front, with the deep surgical clearance distance verified with live US monitoring (Fig. 1b). Resection of the tumor was performed using the elastic needle as guidance or landmark of the deep surgical clearance of 10 mm. The resected fresh specimen is immediately immersed in gelatin solution (Cook gelatin,

Morinaga Co. Ltd, Tokyo, Japan) maintaining original shape and orientation with some thread slings and refrigerated for approximate 5 minutes for solidification using custom made gelatin mixing and processing vendor (HANO Manufacturing Co. Ltd, Fukuoka, Japan) (Fig. 2a). US observation of the solidified gelatin embedded specimen was then performed from the superior surface to assess the entire tumor and its relationship to all the margins and the safety clearance from the tumor invasive front was immediately confirmed (Fig. 2b, 3a). If the safety clearance is felt to be inadequate, additional resection could be easily carried out during the intraoperative period.

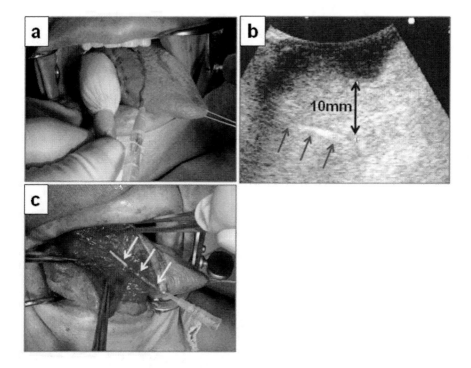

Figure 1. An intraoperative view of ultrasonographic monitoring of a 68-year-old man with squamous cell carcinoma on the right side of tongue (T2N0M0). a) Elastic needle (20 gauge) with a metal core being introduced to indicate deep surgical margin clearance under continuous ultrasonographic monitoring with a 7.5 MHz sector probe. b) Ultrasonographic reflector (metal core) positioned at 10 mm from the deepest invasive front of the tumor. The red arrows show the location of the metal core. c) Resection was performed using the needle (arrows) as the landmark of deep surgical clearance.

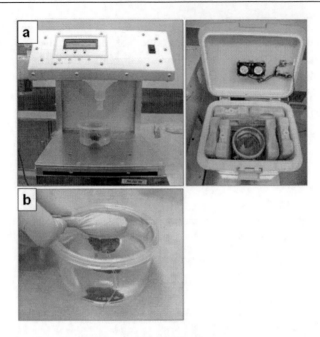

Figure 2. a) A custom made gelatin mixing and processing vendor. (HANO Manufacturing Co. Ltd, Fukuoka, Japan.) The resected fresh specimen is immersed in gelatin solution (Cook gelatin, Morinaga Co. Ltd, Tokyo, Japan) maintaining original shape and orientation with some thread slings, and refrigerated for 5 minutes for solidification. b) Ultrasonographic observation of the solidified gelatin embedded specimen was performed from the superior surface.

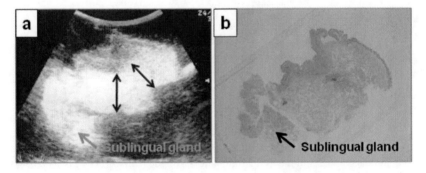

Figure 3. Ultrasonographic image of the gelatin embedded specimen (a) and histological specimen (b) of 52-year-old woman with squamous cell carcinoma on the left side of tongue (T2N0M0). a) The safety clearance of the specimen from the tumor invasive front was confirmed intraoperatively. b) Histopathological section at the same plane of the ultrasonographic image. Excellent consistency between the ultrasonographic image and histopathology can be seen.

Till date, we have already applied this method to 22 tongue SCC patients who had undergone surgical treatment at the Department of Oral and Maxillofacial Surgery, Kyushu Dental College Hospital from 2005 to 2009. All patients were diagnosed with primary squamous cell carcinoma of tongue as T1N0-T2N0 and enrolled after ethical approval from Kyushu Dental College Hospital Ethics Committee. The sex ratio was 13 men and 9 women while the median age was 68.4 years old (range; 38-91 years).The clinical T stages were T1; 6 cases and T2; 16 cases, based on the criteria of the International Union against Cancer (UICC 1997). Then, we compared the tumor thickness of US images to tumor thickness of histological specimens; the mean difference between them was 1.20 mm, which indicated a good correlation and no underestimation in any of the cases (Fig. 3,4). At present, frozen sections is the standard method used to confirm the existence of tumor cells in the surgical margin. Although widely used, it cannot be used to confirm the entire margin. In contrast with the present method, we were able to confirm the safety clearance of the entire resected specimen. High resolution diagnostic intraoral ultrasound works excellently for real time examinations of soft tissues and has the advantages of being non-invasive, radiation free, rapid, repeatable and portable.

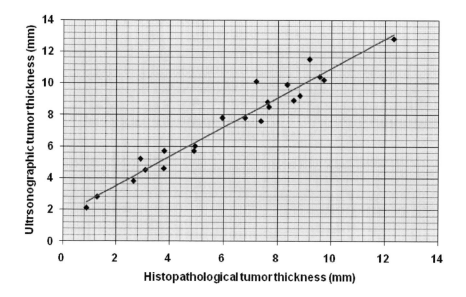

Figure 4. Relationship between the Ultrasonographic tumor thickness and Histopathological tumor thickness.

CONCLUSION

The present method of intraoral intra-operative US was found to be an accurate and reliable tool for assessing tumor thickness and surgical clearance in tongue carcinomas. Further, in near future we believe that this technique would be able to combine less invasive surgery with optimal resection and thus lead to minimal functional disorders of tongue with improved QOL.

REFERENCES

[1]   Ildstad ST, Bigelow ME. Remensnyder JP. Squamous cell carcinoma of the mobile tongue. Clinical behavior and results of current therapeutic modalities. *Am J Surg.* 1983; 145: 443-449

[2]   Silver CE, Moisa II. Elective treatment of the neck in cancer of the oral tongue. *Semin Surg Oncol.* 1991; 7:14-19

[3]   Spiro R, Huvos A, Wong G. Predictive value of tumor thickness in squamous carcinomas confined to the tongue and floor of the mouth. *Am J Surg* 1986; 152: 345-350.

[4]   Rasgon B, Cruz R, Hilsinger R. Relation of lymph-node metastasis to histopathologic appearance in oral cavity and oropharyngeal carcinoma: a case series and literature review. *Laryngoscope* 1988; 99: 1103-1110.

[5]   Sutton DN, Brown JS, Rogers SN, Vaughan ED, Woolgar JA. : The prognostic implications of the surgical margin in oral squamous cell carcinoma. *Int J Oral Maxillofac Surg* 2003; 32: 30-34.

[6]   O'Brien CJ, Lauer CS, Fredricks S, Clifford AR, McNeil EB, Bagia JS, Koulmandas C. Tumor thickness influences prognosis of T1 and T2 oral cavity cancer-but what thickness? *Head Neck* 2003; 25:937-945.

[7]   Kirita K, Okabe S, Izumo T, Sugimura M. Risk factors for the postoperative local recurrence of tongue carcinoma. *J Oral Maxillofac Surg* 1994 ;52 :149-154.

[8]   Looser KG, Shah JP, Strong EW. The significance of positive margins in surgically resected epidermoid carcinomas. *Head Neck Surg* 1978; 1: 107-111.

[9]   Yuen APW, Lam KY, Chan AC, Wei WI, Lam LK. Clinicopathological analysis of local spread of carcinoma of the tongue. *Am J Surg* 1998; 175: 242-244.

[10] Shintani S, Nakayama B, Matsuura H, Hasegawa Y. Intraoral ultrasonography is useful to evaluate tumor thickness in tongue carcinoma. *Am J Surg* 1997;173 :345-347.

[11] Shintani S, Yoshihama Y, Ueyama Y, Terakado N, Kamei S, Fijimoto Y. The usefulness of intraoral ultrasonography in the evaluation of oral cancer. *Int J Oral maxillofac Surg* 2001;30 :139-143.

[12] Yuen APW, Ng RW, Lam PK, Ho A. Preoperative measurement of tumor thickness of oral tongue carcinoma with intraoral ultrasonography. *Head Neck* 2008; 30: 230-234.

[13] Songra AK, Ng SY, Farthing P, Hutchison IL, Bradley PF. Observation of tumor thickness and resection margin at surgical excision of primary oral squamous cell carcinoma: assessment by ultrasound. *Int J Oral Maxillofac Surg* 2006; 35: 324-331.

[14] Natori T, Koga M, Anegawa E, Nakashima Y, Tetsuka M, Yoh J, Kusukawa J. Usefulness of intra-oral ultrasonography to predict neck metastasis in patients with tongue carcinoma. *Oral Dis.* 2008 ;14 :591-599.

[15] Kaneoya A, Hasegawa S, Tanaka Y, Omura K. Quantitative analysis of invasive front in tongue cancer using ultrasonography. *J Oral Maxillofac Surg.* 2009; 67: 40-6.

[16] Yamane M, Ishii J, Izumo T, Nagasawa T, Amagasa T. Noninvasive quantitative assessment of oral tongue cancer by intraoral ultrasonography. *Head Neck.* 2007; 29: 307-14.

[17] Tominaga K, Yamamoto K, Khanal A, Morimoto Y, Tanaka T, Kodama M, Fukuda J. Intraoperative surgical clearance confirmation of tongue carcinomas using ultrasound. *Dentomaxillofac Radiol.* 2007; 36 :409-411.

[18] Kurokawa H, Hirashima S, Morimoto Y, Yamashita Y, Tominaga K, Takamori K, Igawa K, Takahashi T, Fukuda J: Preoperative ultrasound assessment of tumour thickness in tongue carcinomas. *Asian J Oral Maxillofac Surg* 2005; 17: 162-167.

[19] Kodama M, Khanal A, Habu M, Iwanaga K, Yoshioka I, Tanaka T, Morimoto Y, Tominaga K. Ultrasonography for intraoperative determination of tumor thickness and resection margin in tongue carcinomas. *J Oral Maxillofac Surg.* 2010 ;68 :1746-1752.

In: Squamous Cell Carcinoma
Editor: Daniel V. Mortensen

ISBN: 978-1-61209-929-3
© 2012 Nova Science Publishers, Inc.

Chapter 8

ORAL CUNICULATUM CARCINOMA: LITERATURE REVIEW

Yoann Pons[*]

ENT and Head and Neck Surgery Department,
Hôpital du Val de Grâce, Paris, France

ABSTRACT

Introduction. Cuniculatum carcinoma is a well-differentiated form of squamous cell carcinoma that shares histological characteristics with papillary squamous cell carcinoma and verrucous carcinoma. Cuniculatum carcinoma usually occurs on the plantar region, and only few cases involving the oral cavity have been described in the literature.

Methods. A review of the oral cuniculatum carcinoma cases retrieved in the pubmed and google scholar has been performed.

Results. We reviewed 19 cases of oral cuniculatum carcinomas. All of the patients were in a great deal of pain. Clinical criteria, osseous lysis and the coexistence of multiple intraosseous well-differentiated, hyperkeratotic papillomatous lesions with few cellular atypies sign the diagnosis. Cervical and distant metastases were rare.

* Corresponding author: Yoann Pons, MD, Service d'ORL Chirurgie Cervicofaciale, Hôpital du Val-de-Grâce, 74, Boulevard de Port Royal, 75005 Paris, France, E-mail: pons.yoann@gmail.com, Telephone: 00 33 6 89 94 88 39

Conclusion. The diagnosis is often delayed because the histological diagnosis may be difficult. Although cuniculatum carcinoma displays aggressive behaviour locally, lymph nodes infiltration and metastasis are rare. The therapy of choice is the surgery alone, after which the prognosis is excellent.

First described in 1954 by Aird et al [1], cuniculatum carcinoma is a well-differentiated form of squamous cell carcinoma that shares histological characteristics with squamous cell carcinoma and verrucous carcinoma. The cellular elements of the cuniculatum carcinoma are organized into ramified sinuses and keratin-filled crypts, looking like rabbit burrows or *Cuniculatum* in Latin. Cuniculatum carcinoma usually appears on the plantar region. Only few cases involving the oral cavity have been described in the literature [2-10].

The author reviewed the oral cases of cuniculatum carcinoma previously published in the literature.

PATIENTS AND METHODS

Patients

All of the cases previously published in English were found in an Internet database (PubMed, Google Scholar) and analyzed.

Methods

The following data were collected: age, gender, initial clinical presentation, radiological aspect, treatment, follow-up, recurrences and survival. We calculated the mean for each of these categories including data from all patients retrieved in literature.

RESULTS

We collected 19 cases published in the medical literature [2-10].

On average, the patients were 54 years old. The gender ratio was of men and women 6:1.

The more frequent clinical presentation was a painful progressive tumor (8 mandibular tumors, 6 maxillary tumors, 2 hard palate tumors, 1 buccal floor tumor, 1 tonsilar tumor and 1 tongue bas tumor) [2-10].

Tobacco consumption was retrieved in 4 patients [3,4,6], and alcohol chronic consumption in 3 patients [3,4].

Two cases of cervical nodal metastasis were reported [4,5], and one case of lung metastasis [2].

Surgery was performed in 18 of the 19 cases. Post-operative irradiation was performed in one case [3]. Radiotherapy alone was performed in one case [2].

All the patients were disease free survival after a mean follow up of 40 months.

DISCUSSION

There was masculine tendency found for cuniculatum carcinoma in the literature (13 of the 19 cases described occurred in men) [2-10].

In the literature, cuniculatum carcinoma predominantly affects older patients with a mean age of 54 years (range: 9-82) [2-10].

Many possible etiologic factors have been implicated such as Human Papilloma Virus, chronic trauma or inflammation, radiation or arsenic ingestion. However the real aetiology remains unclear [4,9]. Tobacco consumption was found in only four of the 19 published cases and alcohol use in only three.

The patients' main complaint that led to consultation was pain, which was often related to tumor infection.

The patients usually present with a mucosal exophytic lesion or a submucosal lesion with loosening of the teeth, which mimics a periodontal abscess. In one case the lesion remained intraosseous with no mucosal involvement [7]. Bone involvement is typical in this type of tumor.

Upon macroscopical examination, cuniculatum carcinoma showed both exophytic and endophytic growth. The exclusively exophytic form is called verrucous carcinoma. The well-differentiated squamous cells of the papillomatous surface penetrate deeply into the underlying tissues, creating ramified sinuses and crypts that look like rabbit burrows or *cuniculus* (thus the name *cuniculatum*) [1]. The keratin-filled crypts tend to discharge a yellowish, foul-smelling secretion. Microscopical studies found a hyperkeratinized, well-defined tumor with respect to the basal membrane. The mitosis rate was normal or a little increased and the tumor cells exhibited only mild cytological atypia. Therefore, the presence of prominent keratinization, keratin-filled crypts and a minimal amount of cytologic atypies can assist in the final diagnosis of cuniculatum carcinoma [4].

Cuniculatum carcinoma is a locally aggressive tumor of the oral cavity and the therapy of choice should be en bloc resection with free margins and immediate reconstruction when possible. The roles of chemotherapy and radiotherapy have yet to be studied; nonetheless, one patient in the literature was treated exclusively by radiotherapy with success [2].

Although locally aggressive, cuniculatum carcinoma is rarely associated with lymph nodes metastasis and distant disease. Neck dissection should be performed only if the lymph nodes appear enlarged upon examination or CT.

Although only a small number of cuniculatum carcinoma cases have been described in the literature, all studies show that even with the local aggressive tendency of cuniculatum carcinoma, patients could expect a good prognosis once an excision with free-margins has been performed. Among the 19 maxillofacial cases, only two cases of lymph node metastasis was reported and only one case shown to have distant metastasis.

REFERENCES

[1]   Aird I, Johnson HD, Lennox B, Stansfeld AG. Epithelioma cuniculatum: a variety of squamous carcinoma pedicular to the foot. *Br J Surg.* 1954;42(173):245-50.
[2]   Flieger S, Owinski T. Epithelioma cuniculatum an unsual form of mouth and jaw neoplasm. *Czas Stomatol.* 1977;30 :395-401.
[3]   Kahn JL, Blez P, Gasser B, Weill-Bousson M, Vetter JM, Champy M. Carcinoma cuniculatum. Apropos of 4 cases with orofacial involvement. *Rev Stomatol Chir Maxillofac.* 1991;92:27-33.
[4]   Delahaye JF, Janser JC, Rodier JF, Auge B. Cuniculatum carcinoma: 6 cases and review of the literature. *J Chir* 1994 Feb;131(2):73-78.
[5]   Huault M, Laroche C, Levy J, Laxenaire A, Roucayrol AM, Scheffer P. Epithelioma cuniculatum. Apropos of a case in the anterior gingiva with involvement of the mandibular symphyseal bone and reconstruction

using a fibular osteocutaneous flap and integrated implant. *Rev Stomatol Chir Maxillofac.* 1998;99:143-8.

[6]   Allon D, Kaplan I, Manor R, Calderon S. Carcinoma cuniculatum of the jaw: a rare variant of oral carcinoma. *Oral surg Med Oral Pathol Oral Radiol Endod* 2002; 94:601-8.

[7]   Raguse JD, Menneking H, Scholmann HJ, et al. Manifestation of carcinoma cuniculatum in the mandible. *Oral Oncol extra* 2006;42:173-175.

[8]   Kruse AL, Graetz KW. Carcinoma cuniculatum: a rare entity in the oral cavity. *J Craniofac Surg.* 2009 Jul;20(4):1270-2.

[9]   Burkhardt A. Verrucous carcinoma and carcinoma cuniculatum-forms of squamous cell carcinoma? Hautarzt. 1986;37:373-83.

[10] Pons Y, Kerrary S, Cox A, Guerre A, Bertolus C, Gruffaz F, Capron F, Goudot P, Ruhin-Poncet B. Mandibular cuniculatum carcinoma: Apropos of 3 cases and literature review. *Head Neck.* 2010 Jul 27. [Epub ahead of print]

In: Squamous Cell Carcinoma
Editor: Daniel V. Mortensen

ISBN: 978-1-61209-929-3
© 2012 Nova Science Publishers, Inc.

Chapter 9

IMAGING OF SQUAMOUS CELL CARCINOMA

Lorenzo Faggioni[*1], *Emanuele Neri*[1], *Pietro Bemi*[1],
Eugenia Picano[1], *Francesca Pancrazi*[1],
Veronica Seccia[2], *Luca Muscatello*[2],
Stefano Sellari Franceschini[2] *and Carlo Bartolozzi*[1]

[1]Diagnostic and Interventional Radiology, University of Pisa, Italy
[2]Division of Otorhinolaryngology, University of Pisa, Italy

ABSTRACT

Imaging of squamous cell carcinoma (SCC) can be a challenging task and usually requires a combination of several imaging modalities that provide different complimentary information about tumor morphology and characterization, as well as indications about tumor prognosis and treatment planning. In this chapter, the role of the various imaging techniques (such as Computed Tomography [CT], Magnetic Resonance Imaging [MRI], and Positron Emission Tomography [PET]) available for the evaluation of head-and-neck SCC will be illustrated, and imaging findings will be discussed along with their correlation with

[*] Corresponding author: Address: Via Paradisa, 2 - 56100 Pisa (Italy). Email lfaggioni@sirm.org, Telephone +39050997312, Fax +39050997316

pathologic features. To this purpose, modern multidetector CT technology allows an accurate assessment of tumor extent and morphology owing to its excellent spatial resolution and the possibility to perform 2D and 3D reconstructions of native images with voxel isotropy, while MRI plays a major role for tumor characterization due to its superior contrast resolution and its multiparametric nature. On the other hand, PET can provide metabolic data that are useful for detection of disease recurrence after treatment and lymph node and/or distant dissemination. Particular attention will also be paid to emerging imaging modalities, such as CT perfusion, that can provide functional information about tumor vascularity and represent promising tools for noninvasive evaluation of tumor prognosis before chemo-radiation therapy, as well as of early disease recurrence after treatment.

1. INTRODUCTION

Imaging plays a fundamental role for detection and characterization of squamous cell carcinoma (SCC), as well as to evaluate its anatomical extent and the potential involvement of nearby organs for treatment planning purposes. In this chapter the main imaging modalities for SCC will be illustrated, with particular reference to Computed Tomography (CT) and Magnetic Resonance Imaging (MRI) of head-and-neck SCC.

2. COMPUTED TOMOGRAPHY (CT)

In contrast with the projective nature of conventional X-ray (in which image is generated as the result of the total attenuation of a cone-shaped X-ray beam passing through the patient's body), computed tomography (CT) is based on a different image formation scheme. As its name suggests, CT is:

- tomographic (i.e. cross-sectional), as CT images depict slices which are usually (but not necessarily) aligned through the longitudinal axis of the patient;
- computerized, because production of CT images require that raw data be digitized and processed by means of dedicated hardware and software equipment.

CT image is formed by measuring the attenuation of a narrowly collimated X-ray beam that is generated by an X-ray tube rotating around the patient; this latter is positioned on a table moving in the longitudinal direction, either sequentially or (as happens in modern spiral CT) continuously. This way, a series of parallel images can be obtained as a result of the X-ray attenuation of tissues contained in every patient's section, which is proportional to their average atomic number (Z). The intensity of the X-rays that have crossed tissues is recorded by a detector array arranged in the opposite position to that of the X-ray tube. X-ray energy is then converted into an electric signal that is subsequently digitized and integrated with that obtained at further tube rotation angles. The result of such signal processing is an image in which contrast differences among its various points are a function of the different X-ray attenuation (i.e. different Z values) of the tissues and materials inside the slice.

CT technology has seen a tremendous evolution since its introduction in the early 70s, when imaging times in the order of minutes were needed to generate a single image with large slice thickness and poor spatial resolution on the transverse plane [1]. With the advent of modern multidetector CT technology, it is now possible to acquire images with submillimetric thickness and excellent spatial resolution on all three orthogonal planes (voxel isotropy) over a wide longitudinal coverage in a few seconds [2-5]. In the oncological field, such improvements have led to more sensitive detection of even small cancers compared with older CT equipment, as well as more accurate tumor staging and treatment planning. This holds especially true for diagnosis of SCC, which (especially at an early stage of development) are often small tumors that may easily be missed if an inappropriate scanning technique is used. In particular, in the head and neck region (where SCC accounts for 90% of all primary tumors [6]), the use of a spatial resolution as high as possible is mandatory, as the potentially involved organs (i.e. the pharynx, larynx, tongue, nasal sinuses, and the anatomical spaces and bones that separate them from each other) are themselves small structures with a complex anatomy.

Evaluation of soft tissues is facilitated by the possibility to display the various structures by applying to the raw data relative to the attenuation profiles of tissues as a function of the various angular positions of the X-ray source over time (projection data), convolution filters (kernels) that selectively enhance some features of the acquired images. For example, it is possible to apply high frequency filters for edge enhancement of skeletal structures, or low frequency (soft) kernels in order to gain a better demonstration of soft tissues, together with a higher signal-to-noise ratio due to high frequency attenuation [2] *(Figure 1)*. Window settings can also affect lesion detection; to this respect, it has been shown that early T-stage head-and-neck tumors have higher CT density than normal mucosa, and their conspicuity can be amplified using dedicated display windows with narrower window width and higher window level [7].

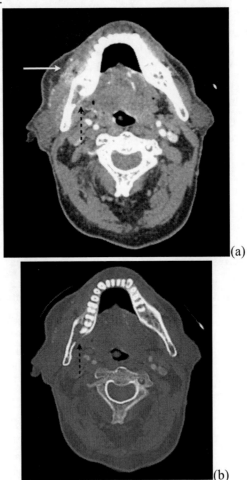

Figure 1. Patient with SCC of the retromolar triangle: (a) contrast-enhanced image with soft tissue window and standard reconstruction filter shows SCC extending to the perimandibular soft tissues (white arrow) and discontinuity of the internal profile of the mandibular bone (black dashed arrow), which is however much better displayed using a bone filter and bone window settings (b).

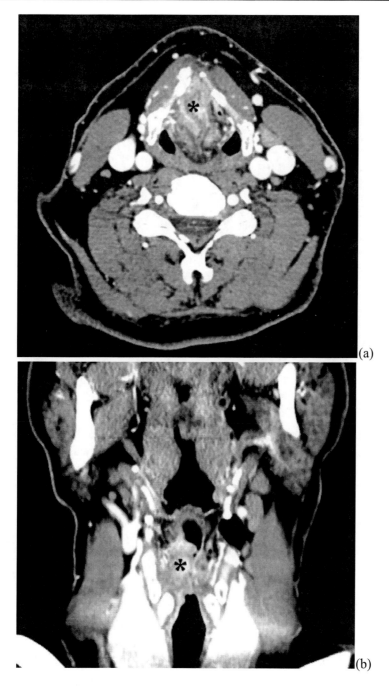

(a)

(b)

Figure 2. (continued on next page).

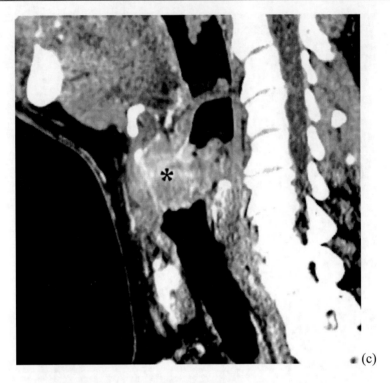

(c)

Figure 2. Transglottic SCC (black asterisk) shown on native axial CT image (a), as well as on coronal (b) and sagittal (c) MPR views.

The choice of a very high spatial resolution (with slices thinner than 1mm) is essential not only for direct reading of native axial images, but also to achieve voxel isotropy for 2D and 3D image reconstructions. These latter are extremely important for the detection and optimal morphological evaluation of SCC growing in a plane parallel to the slice orientation, which might therefore be assessed incorrectly using axial images only. To this respect, MultiPlanar Reformat views (MPR) can be generated, consisting of the geometrical projection of voxels from the axial plane to another user-defined orientation (either orthogonal [Axial, Sagittal, Coronal] or oblique). Such views are useful, e.g. to perform exact and reproducible measurements of the size of a tumor (in terms of distance or section area) either before intervention or in a follow-up setting, as well as to assess its morphology and its potential involvement of nearby structures [2] (Figure 2).

Maximum Intensity Projection (MIP) reconstructions allow to extract voxels with the highest intensity among those aligned in a user-defined direction and included within a given distance range (slab). This algorithm is relatively simple from a conceptual standpoint, requires little computational power (as it only uses a small fraction of the whole information of the dataset), and is particularly powerful for the depiction of hyperdense structures that are continuous over multiple consecutive slices, such as blood vessels filled with iodinated contrast material. To this latter respect, MIP views allow to obtain a detailed reproduction of the vascular anatomy of the territory under investigation [2-5, 8], which can be crucial to assess vascular involvement by the tumor for oncologic staging and/or treatment planning. In contrast with the 2D nature of MPR and MIP algorithms, it is also possible to perform 3D image reconstructions using the Volume Rendering (VR) technique, which retains all the information of the selected dataset (at the expense of a larger computational power requested to workstations) and provides a perspective view of the anatomy by assigning different colors and shades to each tissue, depending on its density and spatial position. VR reconstructions can be important for volume measurements in follow-up studies, as well as to give surgeons a realistic 3D depiction of the territory under examination [2-5, 9-11] (Figure 3).

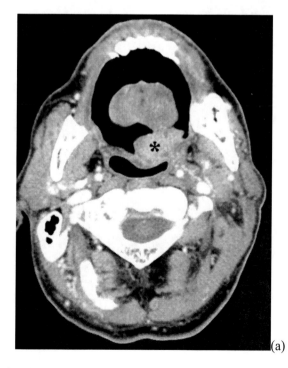

(a)

Figure 3. (continued on next page).

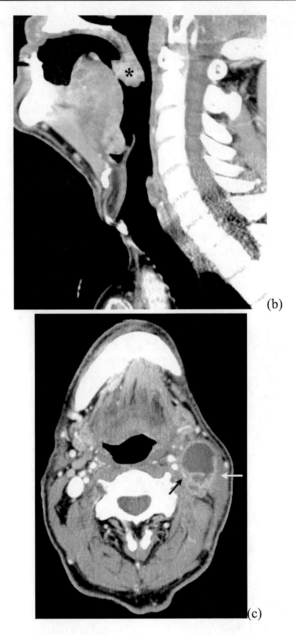

(b)

(c)

Figure 3. (continued on next page).

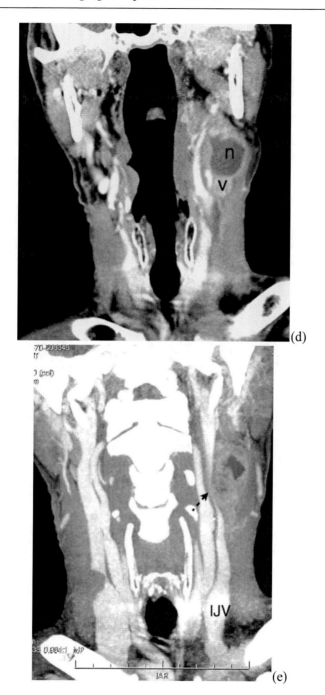

Figure 3. (continued on next page).

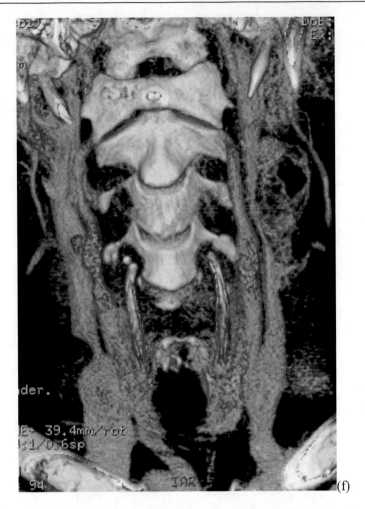

(f)

Figure 3. SCC of the soft palate: (a) axial CT image, (b) sagittal MPR view (black asterisk). (c) Lateral cervical lymphadenopathies with partial colliquation are also present (white arrow) causing infiltration and severe narrowing of the left internal jugular vein (IJV, black arrow). (d) Coronal MPR shows upper colliquated lymph node due to intralesional necrosis ("n") and lower, smaller lymph node with marked and homogeneous contrast enhancement related to presence of viable tissue inside it ("v"). (e) MIP reconstruction shows the entire extracranial portion of the left IJV, including its stenotic part (black dashed arrow). (f) Same view in Volume Rendering (VR) mode.

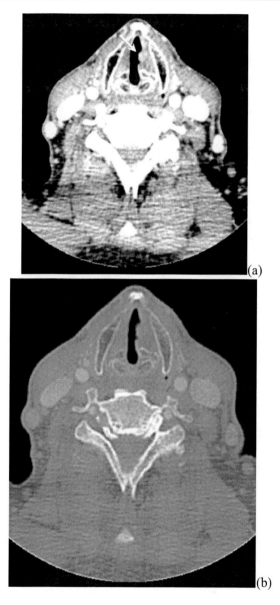

Figure 4. Small polypoid SCC of the left vocal chord (a: white arrow), showing distinct contrast enhancement compared with nearby laryngeal structures. (b) CT image at the same level with bone filter and window settings rules out involvement of the left thyroid cartilage.

Intravenous administration of iodinated contrast material (CM) is another essential requirement of the CT examination for accurate detection and characterization of SCC (as well as of many other cancers). In fact, iodine has a very high density compared with tissues (which are essentially composed of water) owing to its high Z, and if delivered into the blood circulation, it distributes itself as a function of tissue vascularization. In other terms, iodinated CM can be used to enhance the image contrast (contrast enhancement) of tumors and other highly perfused structures (such as arteries, veins, or several parenchymal organs) compared with others that receive less blood. SCC tend to show mild to marked contrast enhancement following intravenous CM injection, as a function of their degree of vascularization; contrast enhancement can be homogeneous or - especially in case of large and/or poorly differentiated neoplasms - inhomogeneous with hypodense areas inside (usually in the central part of the lesion), as a result of partial necrosis and colliquation, while viable tissue tends to be localized at the lesion periphery and may show a ring enhancement pattern [12-13]. Sometimes SCC can also retain contrast in a delayed (>3 minutes) phase after the beginning of CM injection due to presence of a strong fibrotic component, in which CM tends to arrive more slowly [14].

SCC usually manifests as a mass expanding into a hollow organ, such as a polypoid or focal sessile lesion, eccentric narrowing of the airway lumen, or circumferential wall thickening [13, 15] *(Figure 4, 5)*. In more advanced stages of disease or in the case of biologically aggressive SCC, infiltration of the surrounding structures can be demonstrated. In this latter case, intravenous administration of CM is essential to obtain an accurate and extensive assessment of the local extent of the neoplasm, such as vessel invasion, infiltration of perineural spaces, bones, muscles, or meninges [13, 15-16] *(Figure 6)*. Again, accurate reconstruction of the anatomy on multiple planes is essential to define the correct staging of the lesion and indicate the most appropriate treatment.

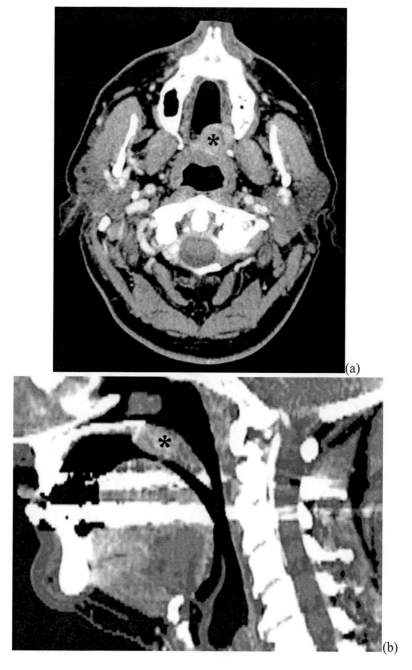

Figure 5. Nodular SCC of the soft palate: (a) native axial CT image; (b) sagittal MPR showing nodular whole-thickness involvement (black asterisk) of the soft palate.

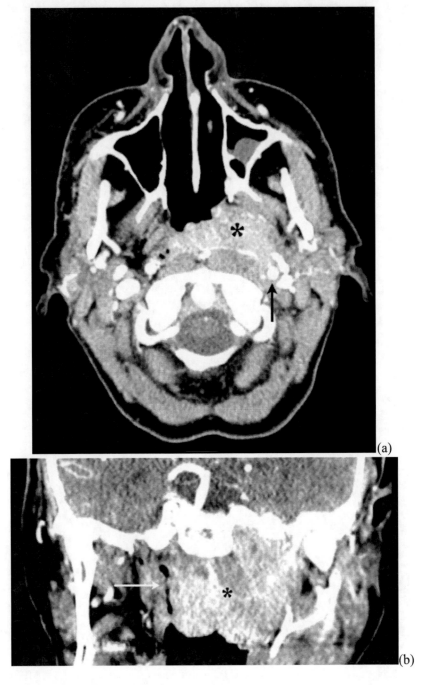

(a)

(b)

Figure 6. (continued on next page).

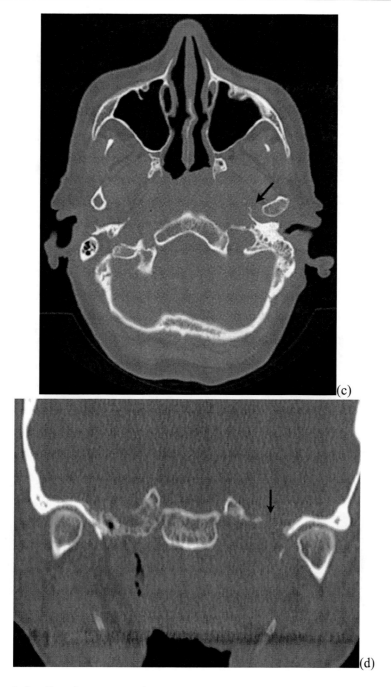

Figure 6. (continued on next page).

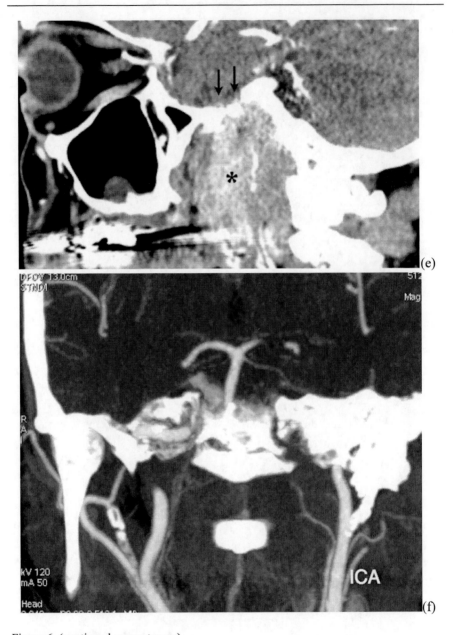

Figure 6. (continued on next page).

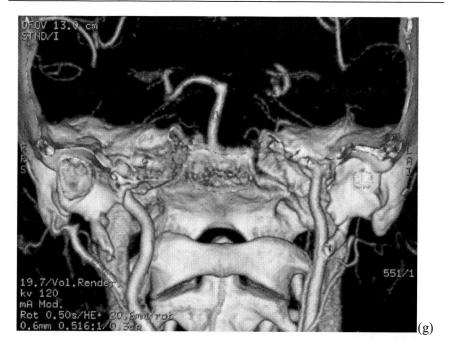

(g)

Figure 6. Infiltrating pharyngeal carcinoma. (a) Axial contrast-enhanced CT image shows large, highly vascularized tissue (black asterisk) protruding into the pharyngeal lumen on the left side and infiltrating the mucosa with contralateral involvement. The lesion extends posteriorly to the prevertebral space and laterally spreads into the deep left parapharyngeal space, reaching the ipsilateral internal carotid artery (ICA; black arrow). (b) Coronal MPR shows wide lesion contact with the left great ethmoidal wing and contralateral displacement and narrowing of the nasopharyngeal lumen (white arrow). (c, d) CT images with bone filter and window settings display bone erosion of the floor of the middle cranial fossa, while (e) sagittal MPR with soft tissue filter and window settings shows multiple focal infiltration (black arrows) of the meningeal involucres. (f) MIP and (g) VR images shows lateral displacement, but no apparent infiltration of the left ICA compared with the contralateral one.

The very short acquisition time afforded by modern CT equipment is a great advantage over other cross-sectional imaging modalities (such as MRI) and allows greater patient comfort, as well as reduced motion artifacts, which in turn improves diagnostic accuracy. Conversely, one major disadvantage of CT is its relatively high radiation dose, which implies an additional risk of cancer that further increases with younger patients. In particular, CT of the neck (e.g. in the case of laryngeal SCC) entails a particularly high radiation hazard as radiosensitive organs (such as thyroid) are included in the scan volume. Of course, the problem of radiation exposure is magnified as patients are required to undergo multiple CT studies over time for follow-up. For this reason, all CT equipment manufacturers have installed dose-saving algorithms on modern CT scanners, that allow to tailor radiation dose to the anatomy under investigation (e.g. smaller patients will receive less dose than larger ones). With automated tube current dose modulation systems [17], patient exposure to ionizing radiation can be reduced by 10-68% on average, depending on the anatomical region, without substantially sacrificing image quality.

Another disadvantage of CT is the use of iodinated CM that, although usually necessary for CT imaging of SCC, is potentially nephrotoxic and may lead to significant worsening of renal function (Contrast Induced Nephropathy, CIN) in patients with renal insufficiency and/or other associated conditions (such as diabetes and congestive heart failure) [18-19].

Although the likelihood of CIN can be reduced by trying to keep the amount of injected CM to the least possible level and hydrating patients before and after CT, the need for CM administration and the relatively heavy radiation burden associated with CT may sometimes suggest to choose different imaging modalities for selected patients, such as MRI.

3. MAGNETIC RESONANCE IMAGING

While CT is a monoparametric imaging technique (as image formation relies on the evaluation of a single parameter, i.e. the different attenuation of X photons by different tissues crossed by the X-ray beam), MRI has the advantage of being multiparametric. In an MRI scanner, protons with non-zero spin magnetic momentum are immersed in a constant-intensity magnetic field and oscillate (precession motion) around their axis at a characteristic frequency, proportional to the intensity of the static magnetic field. Energy is delivered to the protons by switching on an electromagnetic field that oscillates at the same frequency as the spin precession frequency, and image formation depends on the energy interactions between spins and the MR system (relaxation) once electromagnetic energy has subsequently been turned off. In other terms, image contrast in MRI reflects the difference among the various physical parameters that describe the energy exchange in each tissue. For example, it is possible to create T1-weighted images, in which image contrast is given by differences in the T1 relaxation time of tissues, that is proportional to the time needed for spins to recover their initial longitudinal magnetization. Alternatively, T2-weighted images can be generated, in which image contrast reflects differences in the T2-relaxation time of tissues, that is proportional to the time needed for spins to lose the transverse magnetization gained by their interaction with the electromagnetic field.

The multiparametric nature of MRI allows to acquire additional information in comparison with those available from CT, with the advantages of a higher intrinsic contrast resolution and the lack of exposure to ionizing radiation and iodinated contrast media. For this reason, MRI is often regarded as an alternative to CT in patients in whom this latter is contraindicated (young individuals, patients with thyroid diseases or hypersensitivity to iodinated contrast agents), and is typically used as a second-level examination technique for lesion characterization. To this latter respect, the high contrast resolution of MRI can be of great value to define the exact extent of a neoplasm and its involvement of perilesional soft tissues, as it can be able to detect differences in signal intensity that may not be revealed even by contrast-enhanced CT.

MRI protocols for the evaluation of SCC may vary as a function of tumor localization [13, 20]. In general, in the case of head-and-neck SCC, they include acquisitions spanning from the nasopharyngeal dome to the thoracic inlet performed with wide coverage phased array coils, that ensure high and homogeneous signal intensity on the whole field of view with reasonably fast imaging times. Modern MRI scanners with high magnetic field intensity (1.5 Tesla and above) allow to perform imaging of head-and-neck SCC in about 10-20 minutes. T1-weighted and T2-weighted images on at least two anatomic planes are created depending on lesion location, by sending the patient appropriate series of pulses (sequences) that will generate a signal detected by the coil.

On T1- and T2-weighted images, SCC usually shows respectively low and high signal intensity due to its increased vascularization and high cytoplasmic water content compared with surrounding tissues. As in CT, areas of signal inhomogeneity due to intralesional bleeding, calcification, or necrosis may appear and may suggest poor tumor differentiation.

In contrast with CT, MRI also allows to remove the signal of selected tissues (such as fat or water) in order to enhance that of other structures. This is the reason why T2-weighted sequences (on which fat and water tend to have a similar hyperintense signal) are usually performed with fat suppression. This way, only the signal of water will be shown, thus improving delineation of tumor borders and its overall morphologic depiction [21-24] *(Figure 7, 8)*.

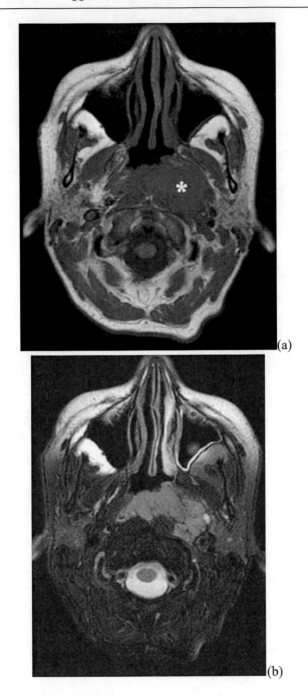

(a)

(b)

Figure 7. (continued on next page).

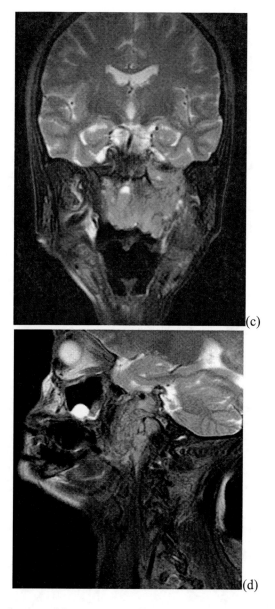

(c)

(d)

Figure 7. MRI evaluation of the same case of Figure 6. (a) T1-weighted axial image and T2-weighted fat saturated images on the axial (b), coronal (c), and sagittal (d) planes. The pattern of low signal intensity on T1-weighted images and high signal intensity on T2-weighted images is typical of SCC (as well as of tumors in general), as it reflects high water content and/or high vascularization of the tumor.

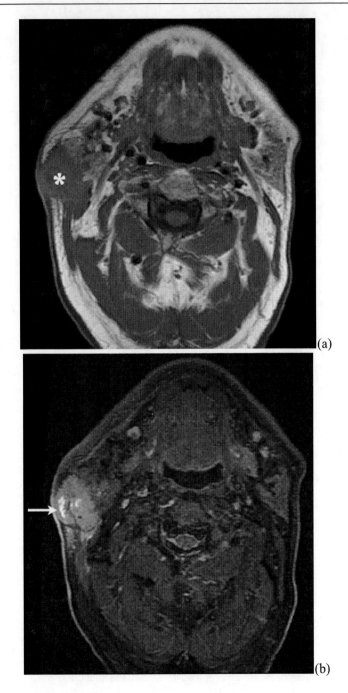

(a)

(b)

Figure 8. (continued on next page).

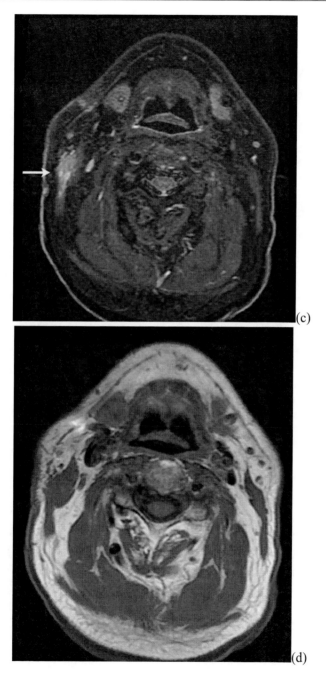

(c)

(d)

Figure 8. (continued on next page).

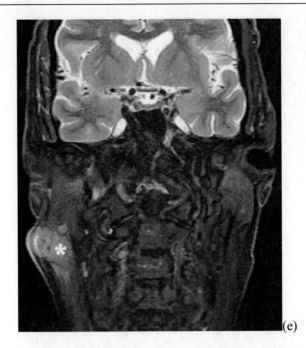

(e)

Figure 8. SCC of the right cheek infiltrating the skin and the ipsilateral sternocleidomastoid muscle. (a) Axial T1-weighted image showing the neoplasm (asterisk) and its relationship with the adjacent subcutaneous tissue, which adheres to it and is thickened. (b) Axial T2-weighted image with fat saturation, showing the tumor with hyperintense (i.e. bright: white arrow) areas of colliquation inside. (c) At a lower level, focal infiltration of the right sternocleidomastoid muscle can be seen on axial T2-weighted fat saturated image, which is not evident on the T1-weighted image (d), but is easily displayed in its entire extent on coronal, fat saturated T2-weighted image (e).

Furthermore, fat suppression is currently used on T1-weighted images obtained after intravenous administration of paramagnetic CM, in order to enhance the signal of this latter. Paramagnetic CM have the same intravascular/interstitial distribution of iodinated CM, but they act by modifying the magnetization characteristics of the environment in which they are distributed. They are considered to be less nephrotoxic than iodinated CM, at least in patients without severe renal impairment (glomerular filtration rate <30mL/min) [25], but in analogy to iodinated CM, they increase the signal of highly vascularized tissues. Therefore, the dynamic behavior of SCC after intravenous injection of paramagnetic CM is comparable to that seen on CT. Fat-suppressed, T1-weighted contrast-enhanced images can be helpful to define the exact tumor extent due to their greater sharpness compared with T2-

weighted images and because they allow to distinguish between tumor and peritumoral edema (as this latter has the same signal of tumor on T2-weighted images, while it has low signal intensity on fat-suppressed, T1-weighted sequences) *(Figure 9, 10)*.

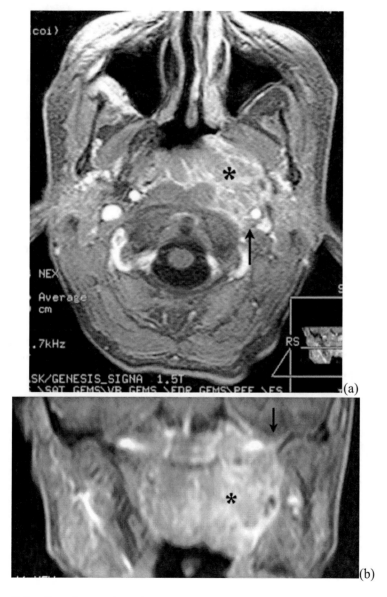

Figure 9. (continued on next page).

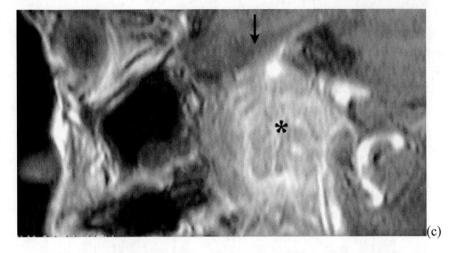

(c)

Figure 9. Same case of Figure 7: fat-saturated, T1-weighted images after intravenous injection of paramagnetic CM on the axial (a), coronal (b), and sagittal (c) planes. Note depiction of meningeal infiltration on (b) and (c) (black arrows) by the SCC (asterisk), appearing as a tail-shaped thickening of the meningeal contour.

Given the absence of ionizing radiation, it is possible to perform a high temporal resolution dynamic evaluation of a lesion by repeating a fast fat-suppressed, T1-weighted sequence several times. This can be important in order to assess the functional status of tumor microcirculation (perfusion), although MRI-based perfusion imaging is still considered to be immature due to its poor spatial resolution and its lack of reproducibility [26-27].

Another peculiarity of MRI is Diffusion-Weighted Imaging (DWI), that allows to quantify the diffusivity of water inside cells. In other terms, water tends to move relatively freely inside the cell cytoplasm in normal tissues, while its diffusivity will be restricted in the case of tumors, which are formed by densely packed cells. DWI can be of value to detect tumor in dubious cases *(Figure 11)*, such as limited SCC recurrence within an area of radiation-induced or surgery-related fibrosis, or small lymph nodes below 1cm short axis [28-30].

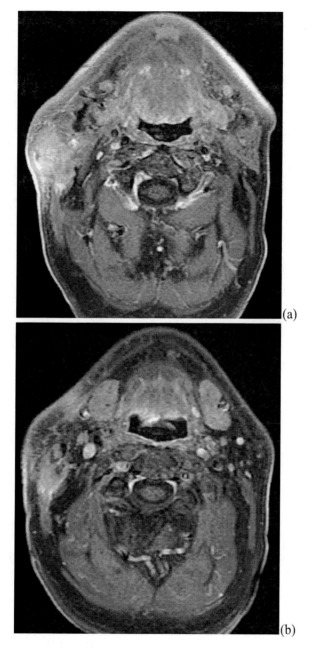

(a)

(b)

Figure 10. Same case of Figure 8: fat-saturated, T1-weighted axial images after intravenous injection of paramagnetic CM at the level of the tumor body (a) and of sternocleidomastoid muscle infiltration (b), respectively.

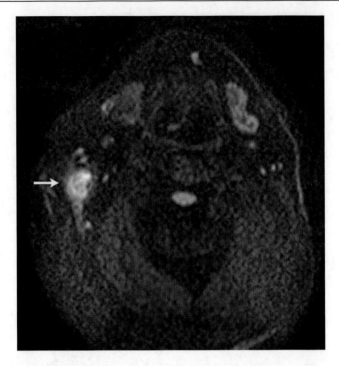

Figure 11. Tumor-infiltrated right sternocleidomastoid muscle shows reduced water diffusivity on DWI image (white arrow).

Despite its advantages described above, MRI also has some limitations. For example, it has a lower spatial resolution than CT (that can limit the evaluation of the tiniest structures, such as in the larynx), and it cannot be carried out in some patients, such as those with pacemakers or claustrophobia. Moreover, MRI is by its own nature sensitive to magnetic susceptibility artifacts, which may occur whenever the magnetic field is distorted (e.g. at the interface between air and bone) and therefore may impair diagnostic accuracy for detection and characterization of pharyngo-laryngeal SCC. In addition, although wide-coverage coils are being used more extensively, it is still impossible to perform tumor staging at an extraregional level due to the need for organ-specific (e.g. head-and-neck) coils to be employed.

Finally, although MRI has a great diagnostic sensitivity, its specificity is still relatively poor for differentiating structures with a high water content (e.g. inflammation vs tumor, or reactive vs neoplastic lymph nodes). Though promising tools (such as DWI sequences) have been developed that may help in this setting, the technique is still too sensitive to magnetic susceptibility artifacts and its spatial resolution is still inadequate, which currently limits its diagnostic accuracy. Other disadvantages of MRI are its relatively high cost and little availability compared with CT [31-32].

4. POSITRON EMISSION TOMOGRAPHY (PET)

Positron Emission Tomography (PET) imaging with 18-fluorodeoxiglucose ([18]FDG) - either alone or in association with CT (PET-CT) - allows to provide functional information about tissue metabolism that can be particularly useful for the evaluation of metastatic disease and SCC of unknown origin. To this purpose, CT images are acquired with a low radiation dose protocol as an anatomical reference and are merged with PET images that contain information about [18]FDG cell uptake (a glucose analog that is interiorized by cells but cannot be metabolized for energy production and therefore accumulates into the cytoplasm proportionally to glucose avidity of cancer cells). [18]FDG uptake can be quantified in a standardized manner and expressed as Standard Uptake Value (SUV), with a high SUV (>5) revealing a high likelihood for cancer.

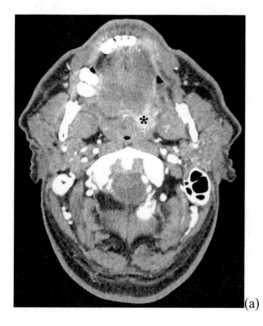

(a)

Figure 12. (continued on next page).

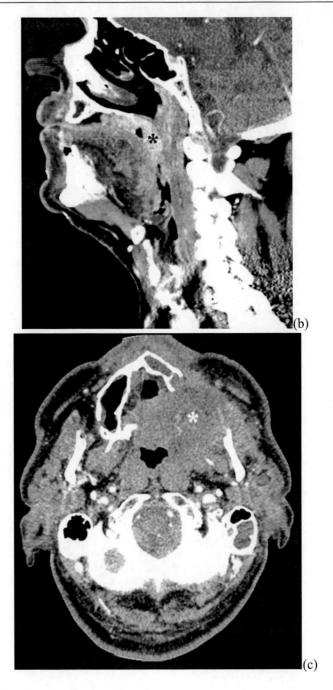

(b)

(c)

Figure 12. (continued on next page).

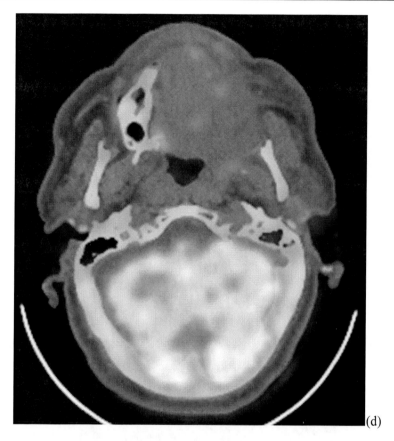

(d)

Figure 12. SCC of the left hemipalate (black asterisk): CT appearance on axial image (a) and sagittal MPR view (b). Patient underwent surgery; on follow-up CT (c), a large tissular thickening with slight and inhomogeneous contrast enhancement is seen in the site of surgical resection (white asterisk). (d) PET-CT ruled out SCC recurrence, as low ^{18}FDG uptake was detected in the area, resulting in a low Standard Uptake Value (SUV) of 2.1.

Typical applications of ^{18}FDG-PET are the evaluation of patients with lymph node metastases from unknown primary tumor, and the detection of residual or recurrent disease after local and/or systemic therapy *(Figure 12)*. Conversely, disadvantages of PET are a substantial exposure to ionizing radiation and a relatively low specificity, which may limit its diagnostic accuracy especially as for lesion characterization [32-35].

5. ULTRASONOGRAPHY (US)

Ultrasonography (US) plays an important role for diagnosis of salivary gland tumors, as these can be easily explored owing to their superficial position. Moreover, US has a high sensitivity for the evaluation of cervical lymph nodes and, in association with Doppler ultrasound, it can be of aid to differentiate between reactive and metastatic lymph nodes *(Figure 13)*. To this latter respect, of course US is also the technique of choice to guide needle biopsy for pathological examination. Nevertheless, it is clear that US cannot replace cross-sectional imaging modalities (such as CT, MRI, or PET) for complete staging of SCC as it cannot provide an overall evaluation of all potentially affected tissues, due to problems related to explorability (deep lesions) and echogenicity (bone/air interface). Another limitation of US is its operator-dependent nature, which makes it poorly reproducible.

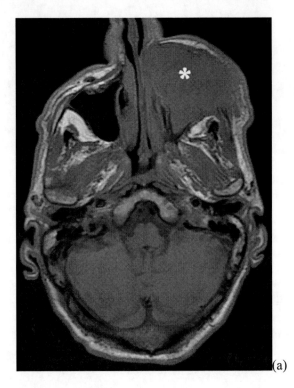
(a)

Figure 13. (continued on next page).

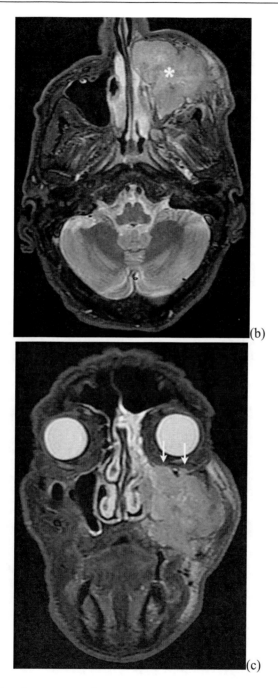

Figure 13. (continued on next page).

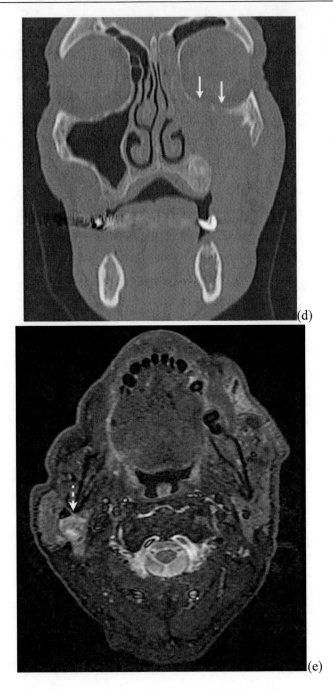

(d)

(e)

Figure 13. (continued on next page).

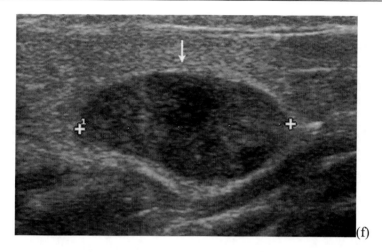

(f)

Figure 13. Patient with invasive SCC of the left maxillary sinus (white asterisk): (a) axial T1-weighted, (b) axial fat-saturated T2-weighted, (c) coronal fat-saturated T2-weighted images, and (d) coronal MPR CT image with bone filter and window settings. Erosion with tumor involvement of the orbitary floor can be seen (white arrows). (e) Axial, fat saturated T2-weighted and (f) US images show enlarged, partially colliquated right cervical lymph node.

6. FUTURE PERSPECTIVES: CT PERFUSION IMAGING

As seen before, CT and MRI play a fundamental role for the morphological evaluation of SCC and the assessment of its local invasiveness (including presence of regional lymph node metastases), which are essential for staging purposes and appropriate treatment planning [6]. However, both conventional CT and MRI can give little or no functional information about the tumor and regional lymph nodes, and in particular, MRI may fail to correctly characterize tumor recurrence, especially in patients having received chemoradiation therapy, in whom the differential diagnosis between tumor tissue and post-treatment sequelae (such as tissular thickening due to fibrosis or edema) may be a challenging task [36-37]. In the last decade, the advent of multidetector row CT scanners has facilitated the evaluation of functional parameters in head and neck tumors, such as tissue perfusion, that can integrate the morphological information derived from conventional CT techniques.

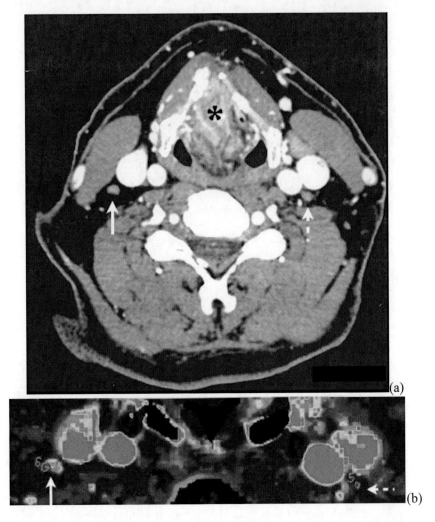

Figure 14. Patient with laryngeal SCC (black asterisk) and two millimetric cervical lymph nodes (white arrows). (a) The two lymph nodes have the same morphological appearance on axial contrast-enhanced CT image, but they have different CT perfusion patterns (b), as shown by their different colors on CT perfusion map (Blood Volume). Indeed, CT perfusion parameters reveal that the right lymph node is metastatic, while the left one is reactive, as confirmed by pathological analysis of surgical specimens.

CT perfusion imaging represents a dynamic contrast-enhanced technique for quantitative assessment of tissue microcirculation, that was primarily developed almost 30 years ago for quantification of cerebral blood perfusion in acute stroke patients [38-39], and has recently been revisited as a promising noninvasive tool for evaluation of the microcirculatory changes of several neoplasms, including head and neck tumors. In this latter field, CT perfusion imaging has been shown to yield promising results, having the ability to differentiate SCC from normal tissues and to correlate with functional or histopathological markers and treatment response [40-47].

CT perfusion analysis is based on continuous recording of X-ray attenuation by a small, fast bolus of iodinated CM over a fixed target region. The dynamic acquisition lasts for a time covering the first pass of CM in the regional vascular bed, during which it has an intravascular distribution [38, 48-50].

The key of classical CT perfusion analysis is the fact that the vascular space of the tissue under investigation is assumed to be comparable, from a hemodynamic standpoint, to a single compartment with one input and one output, corresponding to the feeding arteries and draining veins, respectively. Equivalently, the single compartment model is suitable if it can be assumed that interstitial dispersion of CM is negligible during the first pass [48-50]. If interstitial extravasation of the CM is to be considered (such as in oncologic CT perfusion studies, where CM is expected to leak through highly permeable neovessels), a dual compartment model must be used, provided that data acquisition is prolonged beyond the duration of the CM first pass duration so to encompass at least the initial part of the interstitial passage of the CM [48-50].

Based on a two-compartment model (by which the microcirculation environment can be assumed as formed by an intravascular and an interstitial space, that are in a state of dynamic balance with each other), it is possible to derive the following quantitative perfusion parameters describing the status of microcirculation on a given user-defined region of interest (ROI):

- Mean Transit Time (MTT), i.e. the mean time needed for the CM to pass from the input artery through the tissue microcirculation;
- Blood Flow (BF), i.e. the blood flow transiting from the arterial input through the tissular intravascular space;
- Blood Volume (BV), i.e. the blood volume brought into the tissular intravascular space during the first pass by a given BF over a time equal to MTT;
- Permeability-Surface Product (PS), i.e. the rate of efflux of CM from the intravascular to the interstitial space during the intravascular

distribution phase of CM, which is directly related to vascular permeability [36].

Although relatively few works have been produced so far describing the CT perfusion behavior of SCC, results appear to be very interesting in view of their potential application as markers for both prognostic and post-treatment evaluation purposes.

MTT has been suggested to correlate with the malignant nature of head-and-neck tumors, with malignant lesions (such as SCC) having MTT lower than 3.5 seconds and non-malignant ones longer than 5.5 seconds [44]. Such reduction of MTT has been attributed to the development of tumoral neoangiogenesis with increased perfusion pressure and capillary leakiness [48]. Moreover, Ash et al [47] found a statistically significant correlation between BF and tumor microvessel density as determined after mouse antihuman CD31 antibody immunostaining, and a correlation (albeit not statistically significant) was also detected between BV and tumor microvessel density.

Furthermore, there is evidence [45] that SCC of the upper aerodigestive tract with increased BV or BF are more chemosensitive than other lesions with relatively decreased perfusion parameters, likely due to their increased oxygenation and metabolism. In particular, Zima et al [45] have found that elevated values of BV and BF were significantly correlated with an endoscopically-determined >50% reduction of SCC volume after chemotherapy. Gandhi et al [46] also showed that pre-therapy BV and a 20% reduction of BV after induction chemotherapy are significantly correlated with endoscopic response in advanced SCC of the upper aerodigestive tract. In addition, Hermans et al [43] have reported that CT-determined tumor perfusion rate can be an independent predictor of local failure in irradiated SCC, supporting the hypothesis that less perfused tumors tend to respond poorly to radiation therapy due to their lower oxygen tension.

7. CONCLUSION

Several imaging techniques are available that allow accurate detection and characterization of SCC and are essential for staging purposes and treatment planning. Among those, CT has the advantages of an excellent spatial resolution, fast acquisition times, and widespread availability, which makes it the first choice imaging modality for the diagnostic work-up of SCC. On the other hand, MRI is not burdened by ionizing radiation and iodinated CM exposure and has a higher intrinsic contrast resolution, which makes it preferable in patients in whom CT is contraindicated (e.g. young individuals, patients with renal impairment or severe hypersensitivity to CM), as well as potentially helpful for tumor characterization and the evaluation of local invasiveness, especially when CT findings are inconclusive. PET can provide metabolic information that may reveal metastatic disease or primary SCC of previously unknown origin, while US can find a role for lymph node assessment and to guide bioptic procedures. New functional techniques are emerging, such as CT perfusion, that allow noninvasive assessment of SCC microcirculation and appear to be promising for early evaluation of treatment response, as well as for prognostic purposes.

REFERENCES

[1]   Hounsfield GN. Computerized transverse axial scanning (tomography). *Br J Radiol* 1973;46:1016-1022;

[2]   Faggioni L, Neri E, Cerri F, Turini F, Bartolozzi C. Integrating image processing in PACS. *Eur J Radiol* 2009 [Epub ahead of print], doi 10.1016/j.ejrad.2009.06.022;

[3]   Cody DD. AAPM/RSNA physics tutorial for residents: topics in CT. Image processing in CT. *Radiographics* 2002;22:1255-1268;

[4]   Dalrymple NC, Prasad SR, El-Merhi FM, Chintapalli KN. Price of isotropy in multidetector CT. *Radiographics* 2007;27:49-62;

[5]   Lell MM, Anders K, Uder M et al. New techniques in CT angiography. *Radiographics* 2006; 26 Suppl 1:S45-S62;

[6]   Parkin DM, Bray F, Ferlay J, Pisani P. Global cancer statistics, 2002. CA *Cancer J Clin* 2005;55:74-108;

[7]   Hoang JK, Glastonbury CM, Chen LF, Salvatore JK, Eastwood JD. CT mucosal window settings: a novel approach to evaluating early T-stage head and neck carcinoma. *AJR Am J Roentgenol* 2010;195:1002-1006;

[8]   Prokop M, Shin HO, Schanz A, Schaefer-Prokop CM. Use of maximum intensity projections in CT angiography: a basic review. *Radiographics* 1997;17:433-451;

192   Lorenzo Faggioni, Emanuele Neri, Pietro Bemi et al.

[9]   Fishman EK, Ney DR, Heath DG et al. Volume rendering versus maximum intensity projection in CT angiography: what works best, when, and why. *Radiographics* 2006;26:905-922;

[10] Tomandl BF, Köstner NC, Schempershofe M et al. CT angiography of intracranial aneurysms: a focus on postprocessing. *Radiographics* 2004;24:637-655;

[11] Lell M, Fellner C, Baum U et al. Evaluation of carotid artery stenosis with multisection CT and MR imaging: influence of imaging modality and postprocessing. *AJNR* 2007;28:104-110;

[12] Bongers H, Klier R, Ozdoba C, Lenz M. [The clinical value of contrast CT in lymph node staging in the neck region]. *Rofo* 1990;152:398-404;

[13] Sigal R, Zagdanski AM, Schwaab G et al. CT and MR imaging of squamous cell carcinoma of the tongue and floor of the mouth. *Radiographics* 1996;16:787-810;

[14] Groell R, Doerfler O, Schaffler GJ, Habermann W. Contrast-enhanced helical CT of the head and neck: improved conspicuity of squamous cell carcinoma on delayed scans. *AJR Am J Roentgenol* 2001;176:1571-1575;

[15] Park CM, Goo JM, Lee HJ, Kim MA, Lee CH, Kang MJ. Tumors in the tracheobronchial tree: CT and FDG PET features. *Radiographics* 2009;29:55-71;

[16] Maroldi R, Farina D, Borghesi A, Marconi A, Gatti E. Perineural tumor spread. *Neuroimaging Clin N Am* 2008;18:413-429;

[17] McCollough CH, Bruesewitz MR, Kofler JM Jr. CT dose reduction and dose management tools: overview of available options. *Radiographics* 2006;26:503-512;

[18] Mautone A, Brown JR. Contrast-induced nephropathy in patients undergoing elective and urgent procedures. *J Interv Cardiol* 2010;23:78-85;

[19] Laville M, Juillard L. Contrast-induced acute kidney injury: how should at-risk patients be identified and managed? *J Nephrol* 2010;23:387-398;

[20] King AD, Bhatia KS. Magnetic resonance imaging staging of nasopharyngeal carcinoma in the head and neck. *World J Radiol* 2010;2:159-165;

[21] Tien RD. Fat-suppression MR imaging in neuroradiology: techniques and clinical application. *AJR Am J Roentgenol* 1992;158:369-379;

[22] Lewin JS, Curtin HD, Ross JS, Weissman JL, Obuchowski NA, Tkach JA. Fast spin-echo imaging of the neck: comparison with conventional

spin-echo, utility of fat suppression, and evaluation of tissue contrast characteristics. *AJNR Am J Neuroradiol* 1994;15:1351-1357;

[23] Ross MR, Schomer DF, Chappell P, Enzmann DR. MR imaging of head and neck tumors: comparison of T1-weighted contrast-enhanced fat-suppressed images with conventional T2-weighted and fast spin-echo T2-weighted images. *AJR Am J Roentgenol* 1994;163:173-178;

[24] Ma J, Jackson EF, Kumar AJ, Ginsberg LE. Improving fat-suppressed T2-weighted imaging of the head and neck with 2 fast spin-echo dixon techniques: initial experiences. *AJNR Am J Neuroradiol* 2009;30:42-45;

[25] Thomsen HS. How to avoid nephrogenic systemic fibrosis: current guidelines in Europe and the United States. *Radiol Clin North Am* 2009;47:871-875;

[26] Shah GV, Wesolowski JR, Ansari SA, Mukherji SK. New directions in head and neck imaging. *J Surg Oncol* 2008;97:644-648;

[27] Hermans R, Meijerink M, Van den Bogaert W, Rijnders A, Weltens C, Lambin P. Tumor perfusion rate determined noninvasively by dynamic computed tomography predicts outcome in head-and-neck cancer after radiotherapy. *Int J Radiat Oncol Biol Phys* 2003;57:1351-1356;

[28] Razek AA. Diffusion-weighted magnetic resonance imaging of head and neck. *J Comput Assist Tomogr* 2010;34:808-815;

[29] Vandecaveye V, De Keyzer F, Hermans R. Diffusion-weighted magnetic resonance imaging in neck lymph adenopathy. *Cancer Imaging* 2008;8:173-180;

[30] Charles-Edwards EM, deSouza NM. Diffusion-weighted magnetic resonance imaging and its application to cancer. *Cancer Imaging* 2006;6:135-143;

[31] Lell M, Baum U, Greess H et al. Head and neck tumors: imaging recurrent tumor and post-therapeutic changes with CT and MRI. *Eur J Radiol* 2000;33:239-247;

[32] Alberico RA, Husain SH, Sirotkin I. Imaging in head and neck oncology. *Surg Oncol Clin N Am* 2004;13:13-35;

[33] Chu MM, Kositwattanarerk A, Lee DJ et al. FDG PET with contrast-enhanced CT: a critical imaging tool for laryngeal carcinoma. *Radiographics* 2010;30:1353-1372;

[34] Rodrigues RS, Bozza FA, Christian PE et al. Comparison of whole-body PET/CT, dedicated high-resolution head and neck PET/CT, and contrast-enhanced CT in preoperative staging of clinically M0 squamous cell carcinoma of the head and neck. *J Nucl Med* 2009;50:1205-1213;

[35] Schmidt GP, Baur-Melnyk A, Herzog P et al. High-resolution whole-body magnetic resonance image tumor staging with the use of parallel imaging versus dual-modality positron emission tomography-computed tomography: experience on a 32-channel system. *Invest Radiol* 2005;40:743-753;

[36] Faggioni L, Neri E, Cerri F et al. 64-row MDCT perfusion of head and neck squamous cell carcinoma: technical feasibility and quantitative analysis of perfusion parameters. *Eur Radiol* 2011;21:113-121. Epub 2010 Jul 23; doi 10.1007/s00330-010-1898-0;

[37] Nömayr A, Lell M, Sweeney R et al. MRI appearance of radiation-induced changes of normal cervical tissues. *Eur Radiol* 2001;11:1807-1817;

[38] Miles KA. Tumour angiogenesis and its relation to contrast enhancement on computed tomography: a review. *Eur J Radiol* 1999;30:198-205;

[39] Axel L. Cerebral blood flow determination by rapid-sequence computed tomography: theoretical analysis. *Radiology* 1980;137:679-686;

[40] Bisdas S, Medov L, Baghi M et al. A comparison of tumour perfusion assessed by deconvolution-based analysis of dynamic contrast-enhanced CT and MR imaging in patients with squamous cell carcinoma of the upper aerodigestive tract. *Eur Radiol* 2008;18:843-850;

[41] Bisdas S, Spicer K, Rumboldt Z. Whole-tumor perfusion CT parameters and glucose metabolism measurements in head and neck squamous cell carcinomas: a pilot study using combined positron-emission tomography/CT imaging. *AJNR Am J Neuroradiol* 2008;29:1376-1381;

[42] Gandhi D, Hoeffner EG, Carlos RC, Case I, Mukherji SK. Computed tomography perfusion of squamous cell carcinoma of the upper aerodigestive tract. Initial results. *J Comput Assist Tomogr* 2003;27:687-693;

[43] Hermans R, Meijerink M, Van den Bogaert W, Rijnders A, Weltens C, Lambin P. Tumor perfusion rate determined noninvasively by dynamic computed tomography predicts outcome in head-and-neck cancer after radiotherapy. *Int J Radiat Oncol Biol Phys* 2003;57:1351-1356;

[44] Rumboldt Z, Al-Okaili R, Deveikis JP. Perfusion CT for head and neck tumors: pilot study. *AJNR Am J Neuroradiol* 2005;26:1178-1185;

[45] Zima A, Carlos R, Gandhi D, Case I, Teknos T, Mukherji SK. Can pretreatment CT perfusion predict response of advanced squamous cell carcinoma of the upper aerodigestive tract treated with induction chemotherapy? *AJNR Am J Neuroradiol* 2007;28:328-334;

[46] Gandhi D, Chepeha DB, Miller T et al. Correlation between initial and early follow-up CT perfusion parameters with endoscopic tumor response in patients with advanced squamous cell carcinomas of the oropharynx treated with organ-preservation therapy. *AJNR Am J Neuroradiol* 2006;27:101-106;

[47] Ash L, Teknos TN, Gandhi D, Patel S, Mukherji SK. Head and neck squamous cell carcinoma: CT perfusion can help noninvasively predict intratumoral microvessel density. *Radiology* 2009;251:422-428;

[48] Faggioni L, Neri E, Bartolozzi C. CT perfusion of head and neck tumors: how we do it. *AJR Am J Roentgenol* 2010;194:62-69;

[49] Lee TY. Functional CT: physiological models. *Trends Biotechnol* 2002;20:S3-S10;

[50] Lee TY, Purdie TG, Stewart E. CT imaging of angiogenesis. *Q J Nucl Med* 2003;47:171-187.

In: Squamous Cell Carcinoma
Editor: Daniel V. Mortensen

ISBN: 978-1-61209-929-3
© 2012 Nova Science Publishers, Inc.

Chapter 10

EMERGING NON-INVASIVELY COLLECTED GENOMIC AND PROTEOMIC BIOMARKERS FOR THE EARLY DIAGNOSIS OF ORAL SQUAMOUS CELL CARCINOMA (OSCC)

Joel A. Kooren[a], Nelson L. Rhodus[b],
*and Timothy J. Griffin[*a]*

[a]Department of Biochemistry, Molecular Biology, and Biophysics,
University of Minnesota, U.S.
[b]Division of Oral Medicine, Diagnosis and Radiology, School of Dentistry,
University of Minnesota, U.S.

ABSTRACT

Oral cancer is the sixth most common cancer worldwide ahead of Hodgkin's lymphoma, leukemia, brain, stomach, or ovarian cancers, with about 37,000 Americans being diagnosed annually. More than 90% of oral cancers are oral squamous cell carcinomas (OSCC). While the

* Corresponding author: Timothy Griffin, 321 Church St SE, 6-155 Jackson Hall, Minneapolis, MN 55455, Email: tgriffin@umn.edu, Tel: 612-624-5249

overall 5-year survival rate is about 50%, the survival rate when diagnosed early and treated as localized tumors is as high as 90%. Currently the gold standard for diagnosis of OSCC is early visual detection of a suspicious oral lesion followed by scalpel biopsy with adjunct histology. However, there are multiple limitations associated with biopsies: being invasive clinicians are hesitant to perform them, and patients may not agree to them due to the pain and discomfort of the procedure; the following histology requires expert analysis and is therefore expensive; and issues such as under-sampling add uncertainty to diagnosis. An ideal alternative to scalpel biopsy would be non-invasively collected samples containing biomarkers which can distinguish between oral pre-malignant lesions (OPMLs) and OSCC, and potentially predict the transition from pre-malignancy to malignancy. Methods for sampling and discovering biomarkers of OSCC in a non-invasive fashion have been emerging, including those focusing on whole saliva and cells and other specimens collected directly from oral lesions. These samples are ideally suited for system-wide analysis using genomic and proteomic technologies for biomarker discovery. Here, we describe the current state of the clinical diagnosis of oral cancer, with an emphasis on emerging genomic and proteomic strategies seeking to identify non-invasively collected biomarkers that could improve the early diagnosis of OPML transition to OSCC.

Keywords: oral squamous cell carcinoma (OSCC), oral pre-malignant lesion (OPML), biomarkers, whole saliva, genomics, DNA methylation/ hypermethylation, proteomics, mass spectrometry, sensitivity, specificity

INTRODUCTION: ETIOLOGY, PROGRESSION AND DIAGNOSIS OF ORAL CANCER

Etiology and Progression of OSCC

The genesis of OSCC involves genetic, epigenetic and metabolic changes usually due to insult and injury brought on by carcinogens such as tobacco, and alcohol (Lippman et al., 2005; Sudbo, 2004), and/or viral infections such as HPV (Marur et al., 2010). Generally, the causative insult or injury generates an oral pre-malignant lesion (OPML) which can be a small point occurrence or a field covering a large area in the oral cavity. For leukoplakia, the primary type of OPML, the risk of malignant transformation is between 5% and 17% (Rhodus, 2005; Silverman et al., 1984; Silverman, 2001) with some subsequent studies reporting more variation in these estimated risks, and a higher risk with other types of less common OPML such a erythroplakia (Greenspan and Jordan, 2004). Since most OSCC is preceded by OPML, a primary need in the clinic is to reliably diagnose a transition to malignancy in its earliest stage (Rhodus, 2005).

Current Gold Standard Method dor Oral Cancer Detection: Incisional Biopsy

Unfortunately, even a conventional oral examination (COE) by a highly trained dental practitioner cannot determine if an OPML has transitioned to cancer, or is likely to do so. The current gold standard for OSCC diagnosis is invasive incisional biopsy followed by histopathology (Lingen et al., 2008). Despite being the standard, this method for OSCC diagnosis has a number of limitations. A main limitation to the scalpel biopsy with histopathology is lack of frequent testing of suspicious lesions. In many cases diagnosis of OSCC is delayed, despite patients visiting clinicians, because the clinicians did not biopsy an abnormality they previously identified as OPML (Axell et al., 1996; Lumerman et al., 1995). In fact, a retrospective study found that of those dentists who had diagnosed a patient with OPML, only 14.1% followed the lesion up with a second biopsy within a 3 year period (Rhodus, 2005). Patients are often resistant to invasive procedures such as a scalpel biopsy, particularly for multiple subsequent biopsies which are often necessary for monitoring the progression of OPML. The fact that histological examination is necessary increases expense and effort required to perform a proper scalpel biopsy analysis of a suspicious lesion (OPML or OSCC) further decreasing the frequency that biopsies are performed. Even when a biopsy is performed, lesions which spread over a large area are often require multiple site biopsies which may be taken in a specific location(s) which is not truly representative of the status of the lesion (Rhodus, 2005). The very fact that oral cancer currently only has a 50% 5-year survival rate, when it could be as high as 90% if detected in the earliest stage, is a testimony to the inadequacy of the current standard of practice (Rhodus, 2009).

Rather than histopathology, numerous studies have been undertaken on tissue collected via incisional biopsy seeking to identify molecular biomarkers that could be useful for diagnosis of oral cancer. Some work has focused on detecting chromosomal abnormalities (Reshmi and Gollin, 2005). Beyond diagnosis, many studies focusing on chromosomal abnormalities have investigated their utility in cancer prognosis, and have explored sample collection strategies that are at least minimally invasive (Sato et al., 2010). Additionally, there have been numerous biomarker studies in biopsied tissue using genomic and proteomic approaches (Viet and Schmidt, 2010). Although many of these studies on biopsied tissue have provided new insights into OSCC-associated biomolecules, as clinical tests for oral cancer they all suffer from their dependence on the invasive incisional biopsy, with its inherent limitations as described above.

Current State of Non-Invasive Testing of OSCC: Screening Versus Case-Finding

The limitations of invasive incisional biopsy have motivated the development of non-invasive methods for diagnosing oral cancer. At the outset, it is worth noting that in the area of non-invasive testing methods for oral cancer, there are two distinct types of testing, each with different goals. One type seeks to detect the presence of a suspicious lesion within the oral cavity; the other type seeks to diagnose an already detected oral lesion as pre-malignant or malignant. A recent review by Lingen et al, has defined these two types of methods as either screening (detection of an oral lesion) or case-finding (diagnosis of an oral lesion). Both of these methods seek to maximize the specificity (the ability to distinguish individuals with a condition from those without) and sensitivity (the ability to reliably detect a condition in subjects who truly have it) of distinguishing between either healthy individuals (no lesion), or those with OPML or OSCC. Our focus will be mainly on non-invasive tests for the case-finding of oral cancer which we will refer to as diagnosis, with only a brief description below of the current state of non-invasive screening tests.

A number of methods exist for non-invasive screening for suspicious oral lesions. These tests seek to detect suspicious oral lesions within a population of asymptomatic individuals. These screening methods have been well-described in a review by (Lingen et al., 2008), which we summarize briefly here. The most commonly used test is COE, in which a clinician searches the oral cavity for visible irregularities in the oral epithelium. However, COE has limitations; it can't determine lesions that are benign versus those on a path towards potential malignancy, and it might simply miss small lesions in an early stage of development. Therefore other methods have been developed to improve upon COE. Toluidine Blue (also known as tolonium chloride) is a dye used to stain abnormal tissues, sometimes including OSCC, which would not otherwise be diagnosed by COE. Though sensitivity is high (~100%) for OSCC, specificity is low (~60% varying between studies). Aceto-white methods of screening use a 1% acetic acid solution rinse followed by a visual inspection of the oral cavity under blue and white light. Two commercially available types of aceto-white screening methods are ViziLite Plus, and MicroLux DX. Like Toluidine blue, aceto-white methods are sometimes capable of finding OSCC which might not be readily visible (high sensitivity ~100%), but also makes many innocuous lesions visible and thereby decreasing the specificity of the test. Tissue fluorescence is used in a variety of formats for screening, and case-finding in both diagnostic and prognostic fashions. A major commercially available screening tool using fluorescence-based detection is the VELscope. Studies have reported high sensitivity and specificity, though detection of non-COE apparent lesions is quite rare. VELscope does have utility in detecting dysplastic tissue (OPML) that may extend beyond the location of a visible lesion (Lingen et al., 2008).

Emerging Genomic and Proteomic Biomarkers in Non-Invasively Collected Samples for Early Diagnosis and Monitoring

Studies in Whole Saliva

The availability non-invasive, inexpensive, and accurate tests would foster more frequent testing and improve the early diagnosis of oral cancer. The most prominently used non-invasively collected sample in OSCC biomarker research is whole saliva. This is largely due to several readily apparent advantages (Rhodus, 2005). In addition to being easy to collect in a non-invasive fashion, saliva has direct contact with oral lesions, and can be collected in moderately large volumes (> 1 milliliter) in an on demand manner. Given these advantages, a number of whole saliva-based tests already exist, prominently for HIV detection and also drug monitoring (Kaufman and Lamster, 2002).

Finding new molecular biomarkers of OSCC in saliva is ideally suited for a "discovery-science" approach (Aebersold et al., 2000) using technologies capable of identifying cancer-dependent molecular changes on a system-wide level. For analyses in whole saliva seeking to identify diagnostic biomarkers of OSCC a number of system-wide analysis approaches have been applied. For this review, we categorize these as genomics approaches, analyzing DNA sequence or RNA expression, and proteomic approaches, analyzing the protein complement.

In recent years, genomic-based tests for OSCC biomarker discovery in whole saliva have focused on DNA methylation, mRNA expression analysis, and analysis of microRNA (miRNA) targets, which are seeing increased research interest (Viet and Schmidt, 2010). Although most biomarker studies using genomics have focused on invasively collected biopsy samples, there are still some examples in non-invasively collected whole saliva. In one recent study, (Viet et al., 2007) demonstrated that DNA methylation associated with OSCC can be detected and analyzed in saliva with results at least comparable to that of tissue. A study by (Carvalho et al., 2008) compared the oral rinses from patients with HNSCC to healthy controls. Using a technique to detect hypermethylation, the authors identified one panel of altered promoters which gave high specificity with low sensitivity (90% and 35%, respectively), and another panel of promoters which achieved high sensitivity but with poor specificity (85% and 30%, respectively). Regrettably, no group of biomarkers could be identified which offered both high sensitivity and specificity. However, if biologically distinct paths to OSCC exist as many expect (Schaaij-Visser et al., 2010), then it may be necessary to use a combination biomarker tests that achieve high specificity by correctly tracking a route to OSCC, while having individually low sensitivities. Currently, the limited amount of mechanistic insights into OSCC development makes such an approach prohibitively difficult.

At the level of mRNA expression, (Zimmermann et al., 2007) applied cDNA arrays to quantify mRNA transcripts in saliva from healthy and OSCC patients. They achieved 91% specificity and 91% sensitivity with their panel of four mRNAs indicative of OSCC. In addition, they also tested RNA stabilization reagents to generate a protocol that should allow salivary sample collection in situations where immediately freezing samples might not be feasible. More recently, the same group investigated the presence of miRNA in whole saliva, and their potential as diagnostic markers for OSCC (Park et al., 2009). They found over 300 miRNAs in whole saliva, with two of these showing a statistically significant drop in abundance in patients with OSCC compared to healthy controls.

Despite revealing numerous discoveries of promising OSCC biomarkers in whole saliva, the genomic approaches above do not capture post-transcriptional molecular events that may be associated with OSCC development. These molecular events are best captured by analysis of proteins.

As biomarkers, proteins have numerous advantages, given that they are the biological effector molecules that may be directly involved in the mechanisms of OSCC, and they are amenable to anti-body-based clinical assay development once validated. Additionally, beyond their use as biomarkers, proteins also provide potential targets for therapies aimed at treating OPML or OSCC.

A number of studies have demonstrated the potential of proteins in whole saliva as biomarkers of OSCC. Examples include the proteins interleukins 1, 6 and 8 whose levels are all affected by NF-κB signaling (Rhodus et al., 2004; Rhodus et al., 2005). As a proof-of-principle for point-of-care-clinical assay development, an optical protein sensor was developed targeting interleukin 8 in whole saliva (Tan et al., 2008).

For proteomic studies seeking to discover new protein biomarkers in whole saliva, mass spectrometry (MS) is the analytical platform of choice. For these studies, most prominently "shotgun" MS-based proteomics is employed (Chen and Yates, 2007). Here, proteins are digested to peptides, followed by peptide separations, tandem mass spectrometry (MS/MS) analysis and sequence database searching. The main advantage of the shotgun proteomics approach is the ability to identify and quantify hundreds or even thousands of proteins from a complex biological sample such as whole saliva. For the analysis of whole saliva using shotgun proteomics, separation of the complex protein mixture using two-dimensional (2D) gel electrophoresis prior to MS analysis has been used (Hu et al., 2008), as well as "gel free" separations for increased sensitivity to identify lower abundance proteins (Guo et al., 2006; Xie et al., 2005).

Several recent studies have utilized advanced MS-based proteomics approaches to discover diagnostic protein biomarkers of OSCC in whole saliva. In one notable study by (Hu et al., 2008), MS-based proteomic analysis was used to profile whole saliva proteins from 16 pooled healthy individuals and 16 pooled OSCC patients. Using a semi-quantitative approach based on the number of MS/MS spectra matched to proteins in the healthy or OSCC pooled samples, 23 proteins were classified as differentially expressed. After rigorous biochemical verification in individual patient samples, five proteins (M2BP, MRP14, CD59, catalase, and profilin) displayed statistically significant differential abundance between healthy and OSCC samples. Next they measured the abundance levels of these proteins in 48 healthy and 48 OSCC whole saliva samples; the combined panel of biomarkers provided a sensitivity of 0.90 and specificity of 0.83.

In another study, (Jou et al., 2010) identified the protein transferrin in whole saliva as a potential biomarker for OSCC diagnosis. Starting with 2D gel electrophoresis they identified differentially abundant proteins following up with MS and eventually ELISA verification of their selected marker, transferrin. They showed that increasing abundance of transferrin was associated with both severe and early stage OSCC, and constructed a receiver-operator curve (ROC) with an area under the curve (AUROC) of 0.91+ when comparing healthy and OSCC samples.

Using the MS method of surface enhanced laser desorption/ionization time-of-flight mass spectrometry (SELDI-TOF), which focuses on the detection of relatively small proteins and peptides, (Shintani et al., 2010) analyzed whole saliva from healthy individuals and those with OSCC. Among a number of possibilities, the authors chose to focus on one detected peptide which they determined to be a truncated form of salivary cystatin SA-I. However, it's value as a biomarker is difficult to judge given the lack of reported values of sensitivity, and specificity and lack a study of Cystatin SA-I levels in a larger number of subjects using non-MS-based (e.g. immunoblotting or ELISA) verification.

Although informative, one component lacking in all of the whole saliva biomarker studies above is the inclusion of samples collected from individuals with an OPML. Comparison of OPML patients with OSCC patients is highly valuable, as it would provide insights into which biomarkers may distinguish these lesion types, revealing those biomarkers that may have potential for diagnosing a transition to malignancy early. To this end (de Jong et al., 2010) used quantitative MS-based proteomics to compare proteins in whole saliva from OPML and OSCC patients. For the discovery phase of this study, pooled whole saliva from four OPML patients was compared to pooled whole saliva from four OSCC patients. Among almost 1000 identified proteins, about 200 showed differential abundance between the two patient groups. Based on bioinformatic analysis, the cytoskeletal proteins actin and myosin were selected for further verification, given their known roles in cell motility and invasion for epithelial cancers (Hall, 2009). Western blotting against actin and myosin was undertaken in 12 additional OPML and 12 additional OSCC whole saliva samples. For actin, a sensitivity of 100% and specificity of 75% was reported, whereas for myosin the values were 67% and 83% respectively. Further validation was performed on the exfoliated cells in whole saliva given the potential diagnostic utility of these cells (Xie et al., 2008). Within the exfoliated cells, actin and myosin showed similar differences in abundance between healthy and OSCC patients, linking the results observed in soluble whole saliva to concomitant changes within the epithelial cells.

Studies in Other Non-Invasively Collected Sample Types

One unique and advantageous feature of OSCC is that the epithelial lesion where cancer formation takes place is usually accessible to the clinician. Unlike other cancer types affecting internal organs and tissues, OSCC thus offers the possibility of directly collecting specimens in the form of cells and fluids from the oral lesion. Such specimens potentially offer a valuable sample type for identification of diagnostic biomarkers of OSCC.

One example is cell samples collected by brush biopsy (Mehrotra et al., 2009), which can be performed in a minimally invasive manner. Although the commercial brush biopsy kit is designed for cytological analysis of collected cells for OSCC diagnosis, these collected cells can be potentially analyzed using genomic or proteomic approaches to discover new molecular biomarkers. One proteomics-based study sought to identify protein biomarkers from cells collected via brush biopsy from OPML and OSCC patients (Driemel et al., 2007). The MS analysis was performed using SELDI instrumentation, analyzing 49 patients with OPML and 49 with OSCC. Three peak features in the SELDI MS spectra were found to discriminate the patient groups with an AUROC of more than 0.9, indicating fairly high sensitivity and specificity. Two of these peaks were identified as S100A8 and S100A9; however the third was left unidentified. The use of OPML samples in this study is an advantage, providing evidence that S100A8 and S100A9 are potentially biomarkers capable of diagnosing early transition to OSCC. In a similar fashion, others have measured RNA abundance levels in cells collected via brush biopsy, with one study (Toyoshima et al., 2009) identifying cytokeratin 17 as a potential biomarker of OSCC within this sample type.

CONCLUSION

The move towards discovering new biomarkers for early diagnosis of OSCC is an important step in the right direction towards improving the unacceptably low 5-year survival rate for OSCC. Non-invasively collected samples and analysis via genomic and proteomic technologies for system-wide molecular studies have offered a powerful combination for discovery of biomarkers with clinical value. Unfortunately, despite their promise, initial leads on cancer biomarkers discovered via genomic and proteomic approaches have thus far largely failed to advance biomarkers forward to clinical use (Mitchell, 2010).

So what is needed to provide a successful outcome in the quest for diagnostic OSCC biomarkers? One necessity is infrastructure for collection of large numbers of samples from different patient cohorts, especially individuals with different stages of OPML, different OSCC types (e.g. HPV positive OSCC (Marur et al., 2010)), and potentially longitudinal samples collected along the progression from OPML to OSCC. Coupled with emerging assays for high throughput validation, such as targeted MS-based assays (Addona et al., 2009), analysis of these samples would enable the necessary statistical validation of promising biomarkers to determine those with the most reliability and power for early diagnosis, and those specific to cancer subtypes (e.g. HPV). Another need is better routes for initial discovery of biomarkers in non-invasively collected samples that are truly linked to the cancer progression process. The ability to access and collect samples non-invasively and directly from the lesion site in OSCC provides a unique opportunity to identify molecules directly tied to the cancer progression. Thus, further development of direct, non-invasive sampling methods, such as brush biopsies, that can be coupled with genomic and/or proteomic analyses would be valuable. Results from these studies may guide identification of biomarkers in surrogate samples, such as whole saliva.

Meeting the needs listed above should propel the field towards a new paradigm in OSCC diagnosis, wherein point-of-care devices for saliva analysis (Blicharz et al., 2009) or possibly other non-invasively collected sample types are developed. Such devices would enable cost-effective and reliable diagnosis of OSCC, either in the clinic or potentially even as a home testing kit. The consequence of this envisioned new paradigm in OSCC diagnosis would be a significant increase in the survival rate for this cancer.

REFERENCES

Addona TA, Abbatiello SE, Schilling B, Skates SJ, Mani DR, Bunk DM *et al.* (2009). Multi-site assessment of the precision and reproducibility of multiple reaction monitoring-based measurements of proteins in plasma. *Nature Biotechnology* 27(7):633-U685.

Acbersold R, Hood LE, Watts JD (2000). Equipping scientists for the new biology. *Nature Biotechnology* 18(4):359-359.

Axell T, Pindborg JJ, Smith CJ, vanderWaal I (1996). Oral white lesions with special reference to precancerous and tobacco related lesions: Conclusions of an international symposium held in Uppsala, Sweden, May 18-21 1994. *Journal of Oral Pathology & Medicine* 25(2):49-54.

Blicharz TM, Siqueira WL, Helmerhorst EJ, Oppenheim FG, Wexler PJ, Little FF *et al.* (2009). Fiber-Optic Microsphere-Based Antibody Array for the Analysis of Inflammatory Cytokines in Saliva. *Analytical Chemistry* 81(6):2106-2114.

Carvalho AL, Jeronimo C, Kim MM, Henrique R, Zhang Z, Hoque MO *et al* (2008). Evaluation of promoter hypermethylation detection in body fluids as a screening/diagnosis tool for head and neck squamous cell carcinoma. *Clin Cancer Res.* 14(1):97-107.

Chen EI, Yates JR (2007). Cancer proteomics by quantitative shotgun proteomics. *Molecular Oncology* 1(2):144-159.

de Jong EP, Xie HW, Onsongo G, Stone MD, Chen XB, Kooren JA *et al.* (2010). Quantitative Proteomics Reveals Myosin and Actin as Promising Saliva Biomarkers for Distinguishing Pre-Malignant and Malignant Oral Lesions. *Plos One* 5(6).

Driemel O, Murzik U, Escher N, Melle C, Bleul A, Dahse R *et al.* (2007). Protein profiling of oral brush biopsies: S100A8 and S100A9 can differentiate between normal, premalignant, and tumor cells. *Proteomics Clinical Applications* 1(5):486-493.

Greenspan D, Jordan RCK (2004). The white lesion that kills - aneuploid dysplastic oral leukoplakia. *New England Journal of Medicine* 350(14):1382-1384.

Guo T, Rudnick PA, Wang WJ, Lee CS, Devoe DL, Balgley BM (2006). Characterization of the human salivary proteome by capillary isoelectric focusing/nanoreversed-phase liquid chromatography coupled with ESI-tandem MS. *Journal of Proteome Research* 5(6):1469-1478.

Hall A (2009). The cytoskeleton and cancer. *Cancer and Metastasis Reviews* 28(1-2):5-14.

Hu S, Arellano M, Boontheung P, Wang JH, Zhou H, Jiang J *et al.* (2008). Salivary Proteomics for Oral Cancer Biomarker Discovery. *Clinical Cancer Research* 14(19):6246-6252.

Jou YJ, Lin CD, Lai CH, Chen CH, Kao JY, Chen SY *et al.* (2010). Proteomic identification of salivary transferrin as a biomarker for early detection of oral cancer. *Analytica Chimica Acta* 681(1-2):41-48.

Kaufman E, Lamster IB (2002). The diagnostic applications of saliva - A review. *Critical Reviews in Oral Biology & Medicine* 13(2):197-212.

Lingen MW, Kalmar JR, Karrison T, Speight PM (2008). Critical evaluation of diagnostic aids for the detection of oral cancer. *Oral Oncology* 44(1):10-22.

Lippman SM, Sudbo J, Hong WK (2005). Oral cancer prevention and the evolution of molecular-targeted drug development. *Journal of Clinical Oncology* 23(2):346-356.

Lumerman H, Freedman P, Kerpel S (1995). Oral Epithelial Dysplasia And The Development Of Invasive Squamous-Cell Carcinoma. *Oral Surgery Oral Medicine Oral Pathology Oral Radiology and Endodontics* 79(3):321-329.

Marur S, D'Souza G, Westra WH, Forastiere AA (2010). HPV-associated head and neck cancer: a virus-related cancer epidemic. *Lancet Oncology* 11(8):781-789.

Mehrotra R, Hullmann M, Smeets R, Reichert TE, Driemel O (2009). Oral cytology revisited. *Journal of Oral Pathology & Medicine* 38(2):161-166.

Mitchell P (2010). Proteomics retrenches. *Nature Biotechnology* 28(7):665-670.

Park NJ, Zhou H, Elashoff D, Henson BS, Kastratovic DA, Abemayor E *et al.* (2009). Salivary microRNA: Discovery, Characterization, and Clinical Utility for Oral Cancer Detection. *Clinical Cancer Research* 15(17):5473-5477.

Reshmi SC, Gollin SM (2005). Chromosomal instability in oral cancer cells. *Journal of Dental Research* 84(2):107-117.

Rhodus NL, Ho V, Miller CS, Myers S, Ondrey F (2004). NF-kappa B dependent cytokine levels in saliva of patients with oral preneoplastic lesions and oral squamous cell carcinoma. *Cancer Detection and Prevention* 29(1):42-45.

Rhodus NL (2005). Oral cancer: leukoplakia and squamous cell carcinoma. *Dent Clin North Am* 49(1):143-165, ix.

Rhodus NL, Cheng B, Myers S, Miller L, Ho V, Ondrey F (2005). The feasibility of monitoring NK-kappa B associated cytokines: TNF=alpha, IL-alpha, IL-6, and IL-8 in whole saliva for the malignant transformation of oral lichen planus. *Molecular Carcinogenesis* 44(2):77-82.

Rhodus NL (2009). Oral cancer and precancer: improving outcomes. *Compend Contin Educ Dent* 30(8):486-488, 490-484, 496-488 passim; quiz 504, 520.

Sato H, Uzawa N, Takahashi KI, Myo K, Ohyama Y, Amagasa T (2010). Prognostic utility of chromosomal instability detected by fluorescence in situ hybridization in fine-needle aspirates from oral squamous cell carcinomas. *Bmc Cancer* 10(

Schaaij-Visser TBM, Brakenhoff RH, Leemans CR, Heck AJR, Slijper M (2010). Protein biomarker discovery for head and neck cancer. *Journal of Proteomics* 73(10):1790-1803.

Shintani S, Hamakawa H, Ueyama Y, Hatori M, Toyoshima T (2010). Identification of a truncated cystatin SA-I as a saliva biomarker for oral squamous cell carcinoma using the SELDI ProteinChip platform. *International Journal of Oral and Maxillofacial Surgery* 39(1):68-74.

Silverman S, Gorsky M, Lozada F (1984). Oral Leukoplakia And Malignant Transformation - A Follow-Up-Study Of 257 Patients. *Cancer* 53(3):563-568.

Silverman S (2001). Demographics and occurrence of oral and pharyngeal cancers - The outcomes, the trends, the challenge. *Journal of the American Dental Association* 132(7S-11S.

Sudbo J (2004). Novel management of oral cancer: a paradigm of predictive oncology. *Clin Med Res* 2(4):233-242.

Tan W, Sabet L, Li Y, Yu T, Klokkevold PR, Wong DT *et al.* (2008). Optical protein sensor for detecting cancer markers in saliva. *Biosensors & Bioelectronics* 24(2):266-271.

Toyoshima T, Koch F, Kaemmerer P, Vairaktaris E, Al-Nawas B, Wagner W (2009). Expression of cytokeratin 17 mRNA in oral squamous cell carcinoma cells obtained by brush biopsy: preliminary results. *Journal of Oral Pathology & Medicine* 38(6):530-534.

Viet CT, Jordan RCK, Schmidt BL (2007). DNA promoter hypermethylation in saliva for the early diagnosis of oral cancer. *J Calif Dent Assoc* 35(12):844-849.

Viet CT, Schmidt BL (2010). Understanding Oral Cancer In The Genome Era. *Head and Neck-Journal for the Sciences and Specialties of the Head and Neck* 32(9):1246-1268.

Xie HW, Rhodus NL, Griffin RJ, Carlis JV, Griffin TJ (2005). A catalogue of human saliva proteins identified by free flow electrophoresis-based peptide separation and tandem mass spectrometry. *Molecular & Cellular Proteomics* 4(11):1826-1830.

Xie HW, Onsongo G, Popko J, de Jong EP, Cao J, Carlis JV *et al.* (2008). Proteomics analysis of cells in whole saliva from oral cancer patients via value-added three-dimensional peptide fractionation and tandem mass spectrometry. *Molecular & Cellular Proteomics* 7(3):486-498.

Zimmermann BG, Park NJ, Wong DT (2007). Genomic targets in saliva. *Oral-Based Diagnostics* 1098(184-191.

In: Squamous Cell Carcinoma
Editor: Daniel V. Mortensen

ISBN: 978-1-61209-929-3
© 2012 Nova Science Publishers, Inc.

Chapter 11

OVER EXPRESSION OF P53 AND P21 IN NORMAL ORAL MUCOSA ADJACENT TO RESECTED SQUAMOUS CELL CARCINOMAS MAY BE AN EVIDENCE OF FIELD CANCERIZATION

*Reda F. Elgazzar[*1], Aiman A. Ali[2],*
Ezzat Eldreeny[3], and Khalid Moustafa[4]
[1] Oral and Maxillofacial Surgery, Tanta Dental Hospital and School,
Tanta University, Egypt and Oral and Maxillofacial Surgery,
College of Dentistry, King Faisal University, Saudi Arabia
[2] Oral Pathology and Medicine, College of Dentistry,
King Faisal University, Saudi Arabia
[3,4] School of Biology and General Histology,
Tanta University, Saudi Arabia

[*][*]Corresponding author: Dr. Reda Fouad Elgazzar, Oral and Maxillofacial Surgery Department,
6th floor, Tanta Dental Hospital and School, Tanta University, Tanta, Egypt. Email address:
reda_elgazzar@yahoo.com redaelgazzar@hotmail.com; 00966 508977674 (Mobile) 00966
38574161 (Work) 00966 38572624 (Fax)

ABSTRACT

Background: The mutated p53 and p21 is believed to play a major role in tumorigenesis including oral cancer. The purpose of this study was to determine whether there is an evidence of field cancerization based on the profile of p53 and p21 expression in normal oral mucosa adjacent to restricted squamous cell carcinomas.

Materials and Methods: Immunehistochemistry for p53 and p21 was performed in fresh frozen samples of morphologically normal oral mucosa taken from 34 cancer patients (NC) and 21 non-cancer patients (NN). Stained sections were assessed and the results were analysed using Minitab 13.1 statistical package.

Results: P53 and p21 expressions were found to be positive in 20 (58.8%) and 22 (64.7%) cases of the NC group respectively, and in 8 (38%) and 8 (38%) cases of the NN group respectively. When the results of both groups were compared the difference was found to be statistically significant (P<0.05). P53 expression was found to be higher in the NC biopsies taken from patients with poorly differentiated compared to well differentiated SCCs (P=0.034) and with or without second tumour (P=0.052).

Conclusion: We conclude that the differences in the expression of p53 and p21 in NC compared NN groups, as well as the higher expression of p53 in the NC with poorly differentiated SCC and the possibility of getting a second tumour may be considered as a marker of field cancerization.

Keywords: P53 and p21, Oral cancer, Field cancerization, Second primary tumor, Carcinogens.

INTRODUCTION

Head and neck squamous cell carcinoma SCC represents the sixth most common cancer worldwide [1]. In some countries, head and neck SCC is even the fourth cause of death among the male population [2]. Besides the problem of local recurrences after initial curative therapy, these patients have a relatively high risk of developing subsequent other primary tumors. A yearly incidence of 3-7% second primary tumors cumulative per annum after the diagnosis of a primary tumor has been reported [3-6]. This means that approximately 20% of all head and neck cancer patients will develop a second primary tumor after 5 years of follow-up. Therefore, this condition represents one of the greatest challenges to those involved in the treatment of head and neck cancer, since they exert such an adverse influence on the patient survival [7].

One way to explain the development of a second primary head and neck cancer is through the theory of field cancerization; proposed by Slaughter et al.,[8] (1953) who stated that the exposure of an entire field of tissue to repeated carcinogenic insults, e.g. use of tobacco and alcohol drinking, may render the tissue primed to get further tumor. In other wards, the morphologically non-involved mucosa in patients with head and neck cancer is altered, presumably by carcinogens. Such a carcinogenic influence, if operative long enough in time and intense enough in exposure, produces an irreversible change in cells and cell groups in the given area, so that change of the process toward cancer becomes inevitable. These alterations may include chromosome alterations, gene mutations, and other molecular abnormalities, which may explain high incidence of second tumor in this group of patients.

Alterations in oncogens and tumor suppressor genes play an important role in multi-step development [9] and prognosis [10] of head and neck SCC. The mutated p53 and p21 tumor suppressor genes, are believed to play a major role in carcinogenesis including oral cancer [11]. Genetic alterations in the tumor suppressor gene p53 occur in up to 85% of head and neck squamous cell carcinoma [12]. The p53 functions as check-point regulator, controlling transition from the G1 to the S phase of the cell cycle. p21 is induced by p53 and causes growth arrest through inhibition of the function of cyclin-dependent kinases by integration in the cyclin-cdk complexes [13]. Another role of p21 is induction of differentiation, which is independent of p53 [14]. The inactivation p53 and p21 genes leads to the inability of a cell with DNA damage to induce cell cycle arrest to allow time for DNA repair or the induction of apoptosis [14]. Wild-type p53 may be inactivated by complex formation with mutant p53, viral or aberrant host-binding proteins [14].

Some authors have reported p53 over-expression in dysplastic tissue and normal oral mucosa adjacent to tumour [14-17]. Boyle and his colleagues [1] reported an increase in the incidence of p53 mutation with progression from sever dysplasia to invasive carcinoma. p53 and p21 over-expression has also been observed in non-malignant [15] and malignant lesions [18,19], and in normal mucosa several years prior to malignant change [20]. This provides evidence that p53 and p21 mutation may be an early event in the pathogenesis of head and neck SCC. The question is; could it be possible to employ p53 and p21 profile in normal oral mucosa as a marker of field cancerization and subsequently, predict a second primary tumor?

The mutated p53 and p21 gene products are more stable than the wild-types and can be demonstrated in tissue sections [21]. Therefore, this immunohisto-chemical study was designed to determine whether there is evidence of field cancerization based on the profile of p53 and p21 expression in normal oral mucosa.

Objectives

The main objectives of this paper are to:

[1] Determine whether there is evidence of field cancerization based on the profile of p53 and p21 expression in fresh frozen normal oral mucosa taken from cancer compared to non-cancer patients.
[2] Study the correlation between p53 and p21 expression profile in normal oral mucosa and their possible correlation with the patients' clinical variables.

MATERIAL AND METHODS

Patients and Biopsies

This study was carried out in Dundee Dental Hospital and School, Scotland, with the approval of the Tayside Ethical Committee, in conjunction with Tanta Dental Hospital and School, Egypt. The materials of this study consisted of frozen sections of morphologically normal oral mucosa taken from 34 cancer patients (NC) (Figures 1 and 2) and 21 Non-cancer patients (NN). NC specimens were removed from the wound margin that was left following excision of the tumor. In each case, the tumor had been confirmed as a squamous cell carcinoma following routine histopathological reporting. Furthermore, such lesions were always excised with at least 1-cm margin of clinically normal oral mucosa and all spacemen were confirmed normal using hematoxylin and eosin stain (HE).

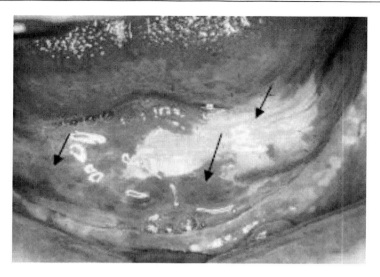

Figure 1. Intraoral photograph showing SCC in Floor of the mouth and signs of some risk factors (arrows).

NN specimens were obtained either as redundant tissue (e.g., during removal of impacted teeth), or from volunteers. Then, all specimens were placed immediately in saline then labeled and taken to the laboratory to be frozen immediately in liquid nitrogen/isopentane prior to storage in liquid nitrogen till required.

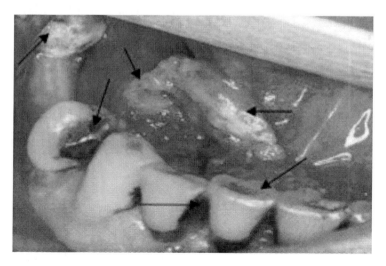

Figure 2. Intraoral photograph showing field change in the floor of the mouth (arrows).

Antibodies

Proteins were detected in the frozen tissue sections as follows:

[1] p53 protein with the monoclonal antibody D07, 1: 50 dilution (Novocastra, Laboratories Ltd, UK), generated against recombinant p53 protein, and specific for both human wild and mutant forms of the p53 protein.

[2] p21^{WAFI} by p21 mouse monoclonal antibody, 1:50 dilution, (Ab-1; Oncogene Science) raised against recombinant human p21^{WAFI} protein.

Immunostaining

Blocks were removed from the liquid nitrogen and 5-µm sections were cut (using a cryostat) onto slides pre-coated with APES (3-Aminopropyl Triethoxy-Silane) then fixed in acetone for 6 minutes. Frozen sections required no pre-treatment. Endogenous peroxidase activity was blocked using 3% hydrogen peroxide in phosphate buffered saline (PBS) for 30 min and washing in PBS for 10 min, then, sections were incubated for 20 min in 5% normal goat serum in PBS, and washed in PBS for 10 min, Afterwards, they were incubated with a mono-clonal mouse antibody against human p53 and p21 proteins for 1 hour at room temperature. Negative controls were performed for each specimen by the omission of the primary antibodies and positive controls by staining sections of a p53 and p21 over-expressing tumor.

Antibodies were visualised with the appropriate biotinylated secondary antibody (Vector Laboratories Ltd, Peterborough, England) followed by the Elite avidin-biotin complex (ABC) amplification kit (Vector) and incubation with diaminobenzidine substrate (Sigma) resulting in a brown reaction product and finally, slightly counterstained with haematoxylin.

Evaluation of p53 and p21 expression

Brown nuclear staining was regarded as being p53 or p21 positive. Sections with ≥5% brown cells were considered positive. The number of stained and non-stained cells was recorded separately and coded as non-stained [0-4], mild [from 5 to 15% of cells], moderate [from 16 to 30% of cells] and severe [more than 31% of cells]. To determine the proportion of positively stained cells, each specimen was assessed by counting all nucleated cells in fields of full thickness epithelium until at least 500 cells had been counted. The percentage was computed for each section for each antibody (p53 and p21).

Statistical Analysis

Stained sections were assessed and the results were analysed using Minitab 13.1 statistical package. As the results were not normally distributed, Non-parametric tests were employed to study correlations and differences between all variables. Mann-Whitney Test was used to compare the expression of both antibodies in both groups (NN and NC). Mood's Median Test was used to study the correlation between the expression of p53 and p21 in relation to the clinical variables in both groups. Pearson Correlation Test was used to evaluate the correlation between the expression of p53 and p21 and age of the patients in both groups.

RESULTS

This study included 2 groups; the 1st one contained 34 patients with SCC, mean age 66.9 years (S.D. 11.4), the male: female ratio was 1.8:1. Biopsies of this group included 25 and 9 non-keratinized and keratinized oral mucosa respectively. The 2nd group contained 21 volunteers, mean age 24 years (S.D. 8.8), the male: female ratio was 1: 2.5, and included 7 and 4 non-keratinized and keratinized oral mucosa respectively.

Fifty percent of the NC patients were tobacco and alcohol users. In the same group, seven patients had non-differentiated SCCs while 27 patients had well differentiated SCCs. Furthermore, 9 patients (26.5%) of this group developed a second tumor.

In the NC group, p53 and p21 expressions were found to be positive in 20 (58.8%) and 22 (64.7%) cases respectively; and the average percentages of the stained nuclei (intensity) among all specimens of the same group were found to be 15.5% and 15.7% for both antibodies respectively (Table 1). Whereas, in the NN group, p53 and p21 expressions were found to be positive in only 8

(38%) for each antibody, and the intensity was found to be 5.1% and 5.4% for both antibodies respectively. When the two groups were compared with respect to the number of positive cases and the intensity, the differences were found to be statistically significant for both p53 and p21 (P<0.05). However, there was no correlation between the expression profile of p53 and p21 in the NC and NN groups (Table 1).

Expression of p21 was mainly detected in the supra-basal and sometimes in the superficial layers of the oral mucosa in both groups (Figures 5 and 6) while p53 was mainly detected in the basal layer and sometimes in the supra-basal layers in both groups (Figures 3 and 4).

Differences in intensity of expression of p53 in the NC patients with well differentiated versus non-differentiated SCCs and with versus without second tumors were found to be statistically significant (P=0.034, and P=0.052) respectively (Tables 2 and 3), however, differences in the expression of p21 between the same patient groups were found to be statistically non-significant. Biopsies taken from alcohol and tobacco users did not show statistical significance in relation to expression of p53 and p21 (P>0.05).

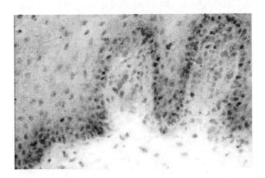

Figure 3. Microphotograph x65 showing P53 expression in NN oral mucosa.

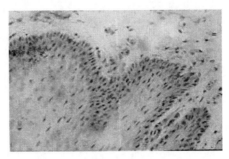

Figure 4. Microphotograph x65 showing P53 expression in NC oral mucosa.

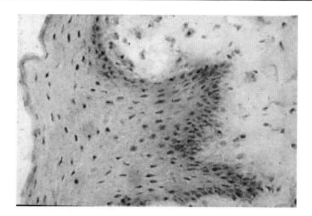

Figure 5. Microphotograph x65 showing P21 expression in NN oral mucosa.

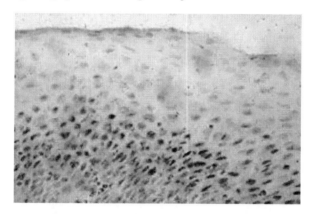

Figure 6. Microphotograph x100 showing P21 expression in NC oral mucosa.

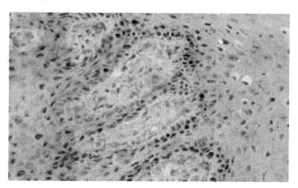

Figure 7. Microphotograph (40x) showing P53 expression in NC oral mucosa with slight dysplasia.

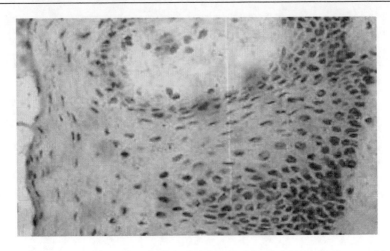

Figure 8. Microphotograph (40x) showing P21 expression in NC oral mucosa with slight dysplasia.

Table 1. The patient data, p53 and p21 expression in biopsies taken from both groups

| | No | P53 | | | | | P21 | | | | |
		Mild	Moderate	Severe	Total	Intensity	Mild	Moderate	Severe	Total	Intensity
GI (NC)	34	4 (11.7%)	11 (32.3%)	5 (14.7%)	20 (58.8%)	15.5%	5 (14.7%)	10 (29.4%)	7 (20.6%)	22 (64.7%)	15.7%
GII (NN)	21	7 (33.3%)	1 (4.8%)	0 (0%)	8 (38%)	5.4%	7 (33.3%)	1 (4.8%)	0 (0%)	8 (38%)	5.1%

Table 2. The median intensity of expression of p53 and p21 in biopsies taken from patients with well differentiated and non-differentiated tumors (NC group)

	Intensity of expression of P53	Intensity of expression of P21
With well differentiated tumor	10%	7%
With non-differentiated tumor	23%	21%
P – value	0.034	0.203

Slaughter et al., [8] proposed the concept of field cancerization in patients with squamous cell carcinoma of the head and neck and discussed its clinical significance for the development of second primary tumors and local recurrences. Since then, the term has been used to describe multiple patches of pre-malignant disease, a higher-than-expected prevalence of multiple local second primary tumors, and the presence of synchronous distant tumors within the upper aerodigestive tract [22].

Table 3. The median intensity of expression of p53 and p21 in biopsies taken from patients with or without second tumors (NC group)

	Intensity of expression of P53	Intensity of expression of P21
With second tumor	10%	10%
Without second tumor	30%	20%
P - value	0.052	0.697

DISCUSSION

Previous studies addressed p53 and p21 as a negative regulator of cell cycle and play a crucial rule in head and neck tumorigenesis [11,18, 22]. Other studies [14] and ours showed that there was different patterns of p53 expression in NC compared to NN groups and that the proportion of cases with positive p53 expression increased in NC compared to NN group. Homann, et al. [5] investigated p53 expression in tumor-distant epithelia and in the corresponding primary tumors of 105 head and neck cancer patients by immunohistochemistry on frozen sections; they reported that over expression of p53 in tumor-distant epithelia was found in 49 patients (46.7%; while in the present study was 58.8%), and it was independent of the p53 protein status of the primary tumor, local primary recurrences, lymph node or distant metastases, or overall survival. Most importantly, they added that mucosal p53 over expression, but not over expression in the primary tumors, was significantly associated with an increased incidence of second primary carcinomas (P=0.0001; while in the present study was found to be 0.052). Brennan et al. [18], reported positive correlation between tobacco smoking, alcohol drinking and the over-expression of p53 protein in paraffin SCC sections; yet, the present study did not prove this relation in the pre-tumor normal mucosa.

Our study confirms the results of Csuka et al., [14] who investigated the expression of p53 in 153 normal pre-tumoral oral mucosa specimens and reported that 11% of the cases showed p53 mutations. On contrary to our results, some authors [23] reported negative expression of p53 in normal oral mucosa; this is probably due to differences in the methodology [24] or because most of these studies were based on formalin fixed paraffin impeded sections where as the antigen expression may be affected by the method of the unmasking techniques [25] or because the antigen in the fresh frozen tissue (as in the case of this study) is more sensitive than in the treated paraffin tissue [26]. In agreement with other studies [18, 25], the present study showed that the expression of p53 was concentrated in the basal epithelial layer whereas p21 was mainly detected in the supra-basal and superficial layers. In consistence with the results reported by van Oijen et al., [27] we could not prove correlation between the expression of both p21 and p53, this is probably because p21 can be activated by pathways (e.g. growth factors) other than the p53-dependent one [28].

The results of the current study reinforce the hypothesis of field cancerization, the view that the remaining mucosa of cancer patients is at risk of getting further tumor. This assumption is supported by our previous studies on the angiogenic profile of normal mucosa in cancer and non-cancer patients [29, 30]. Therefore, based on this and other studies, dietary advice and alternative means of prevention or gene therapy that can affect the entire head and neck region may be of benefit to such patients. We conclude that oral SCC (particularly the moderate and poorly differentiated ones) may induce a field change in the neighbouring morphologically normal mucosa which is reflected on the expression of p53 and p21 proteins, and this may help predict the biological potential of oral SCC as well as the probability of getting a second primary tumor.

REFERENCES

[1]   Ogden, GR, Cowpe, JG, and Green, MW. Detection of field change in oral cancer using oral exfoliative cytologic study. *Cancer* 1991: 1:1611-1615.

[2]   Ha PK, Califano JA. The molecular biology of mucosal field cancerization of the head and neck. *Crit Rev Oral Biol Med*. 2003: 14:363-369.

[3]   Cooper JS, Pajak TF, Rubin P, Tupchong L, Brady LW, Leibel SA, Laramore GE, Marcial VA, Davis LW, Cox JD. Second malignancies in patients who have head and neck cancer: incidence, effect on survival

and implications based on the RTOG experience. *Int J Radiat Oncol Biol Phys*. 1989: 17, 449-456.

[4]   el-Deiry WS, Tokino T, Waldman T, Oliner JD, Velculescu VE, Burrell M, Hill DE, Healy E, Rees JL, Hamilton SR. Topological control of p21 expression in normal and neoplastic tissues. Cancer Res. 1995: 55: 2910-2919.

[5]   Homann N, Nees M, Conradt C, Dietz A, Weidauer H, Maier H, Bosch FX. Overexpression of p53 in tumor-distant epithelia of head and neck cancer patients is associated with an increased incidence of second primary carcinoma. *Clin Cancer Res*. 2001: 7: 290-196.

[6]   Lane DP, Lu X, Hupp T, Hall PA. The role of p53 protein in the apoptotic response. *Philos Trans R Soc Lond B Biol Sci.* 1994: 30: 277-280.

[7]   Ogden GR, Chisholm DM, Kiddie Ra, Lane DP. P53 protein in odontogenic cysts: increased expression in some odontogenic keratocysts. *J Clin Pathol* 1992: 45: 1007-1010.

[8]   Slaughter, DP, Southwick, HW, and Smejkal, W. Field cancerization in oral stratified squamous epithelium. *Cancer*, 1953; 6: 963-968.

[9]   Ogden GR, Lane DP, Chisholm DM. p53 expression in dyskeratosis congenital: a marker for oral premalilgnancy? *J Clin Pathol* 1993: 46: 169-70.

[10] Hill C, Doyon F, Benhamou E. Mortality from cancer in France. Changes between 1950 and 1989 in the population aged 35-64. *Presse Med.* 1992 Jul 4-11; 21 (25): 1150-3.

[11] Sugerman, PB, Joseph, BK, and Savage, NW. Review article: The role of oncogenes, tumor suppressor genes and growth factors in oral squamous cell carcinoma: a case of apoptosis versus proliferation. *Oral Diseases* 1995; 1: 172-188.

[12] Boyle JO, Hakim J, Koch W, van der Riet P, Hruban RH, Roa RA, Correo R, Eby YJ, Ruppert JM, Sidransky D. The incidence of p53 mutations increases with progression of head and neck cancer. *Cancer Res* 1993; 53: 4477-4480.

[13] Franco EL, Kowalski LP, Kanda JL. Risk factors for second cancers of the upper respiratory and digestive systems: a case control study. *J clin Epidemiol* 1991; 7: 615-625.

[14] Csuka O, Olasz J, Juhasz A, Hargitai A, Remenar E, Kasler M. Genetic marker analysis in head and neck cancer. *Magy Onkol.* 2001; 45:161-167.

[15] Dowell SP and Ogden GR. The use of antigen retrieval for immunohistochemical detection of p53 over-expression in malignant and benign oral mucosa: a cautionary note. *J Oral Pathol Med* 1996: 25: 60-64.

[16] Parkin DM, Stjernsward J, Muir CS. *Bull WHO* 1984, 62, 163 -182.

[17] Shin DM, Kim J, Ro Jy, Hirrelman J, Roth JA, Hong WK. Activation of p53 gene expression in premalignant lesions during head and neck tumorigenesis. *Cancer Res* 1994; 54:321-326.

[18] Brennan JA, Boyle JO, Koch WM, Goodman SN, Hruban RH, Eby YJ, Couch MJ, Forastiere AA, Sidransky D. Association between cigarette smoking and mutation of the p53 gene in squamous cell carcinoma of the head and neck. *N Engl J Med*. 1995; Suppl 529: 237-240.

[19] Chang KW, Lin SC, Kwan PC, and Wong YK. Association of aberrant p53 and p21 (WAF1) immnoreactivity with the outcome of oral verrucous leukoplakia in Taiwan. *J Oral Pathol Med.* 2000; 29: 56-62.

[20] Macfarlane GJ, McCredie M, Pompe-Kirn V., Sharpe L, Coates M. Second cancers occurring after cancers of the mouth and pharynx: data from three population-based registries in Australia, Scotland and Slovenia. Oral Oncol, *Eur J Cancer* 1995; 31B: 315-318.

[21] Nees M, Homann N, Discher H, Andl T, Enders C, Herold-Mende C, Schuhmann A, Bosch FX. Expression of mutated p53 occurs in tumor-distant epithelia of head and neck cancer patients: a possible molecular basis for development of multiple tumors. *Cancer Res* 1993; 46: 169-70.

[22] Gartel, AL, Serfas MS, Tyner AL. p21-negative regulator of the cell cycle. *Proc Soc Exp Biol Med* 1996; 213: 138-149.

[23] Papadimttrakopoulou, VA, Shin DM, Hong WK. Molecular and cellular biomarkers for field cancerization and multistep process in head and neck tumorigenesis. *Cancer Metastasis Rev* 1996; 15: 53-76.

[24] El-Gazzar RF, Macluskey M, Ogden GR. The effect of the antibody used and method of quantification on oral mucosal vascularity. *Int J Oral Maxillofac Surg*. 2005 May 2.

[25] Gusterson BA, Anbazhagan R, Warren W, Midgely C, Lane DP, O'Hare M, Stamps A, Carter R, Jayatilake H.. Expression of p53 in pre-malignant and malignant squamous epithelium. *Oncogene* 1991; 6: 1785-1789.

[26] Kropveld, A, van Mansfeld, ADM, Nabben, N, Hordijk, GJ, and Slootweg, PJ. Discordance of p53 status in matched primary tumors and metastases in head and neck squamous cell carcinoma patients. Oral Oncol, *Eur J Cancer* 1996; 32B: 388-393.

[27] van Oijen, Tilanus, MGJ, Medema, RH, and Slootweg, PJ: expression of p21 (Waf1/Cip1) in head and neck cancer in relation to proliferation, differentiation, p53 status and cyclin D1 expression. *J Oral Pathol Med* 1998: 27: 367-75.

[28] Hiranuma H, Jikko A, Maeda T, Matumura S, Murakami S, and Fukuda Y. An analysis of the prognostic significance of p53 status for squamous cell carcinoma of the oral cavity treated by radiotherapy. *Oral Oncology* 1998: 34: 513-518.

[29] El-Gazzar R, Macluskey M, Ogden GR. Evidence for a field change effect based on angiogenesis in the oral mucosa? A brief report. *Oral Oncol.* 2005 Jan;41(1):25-30.

[30] El-Gazzar R, Macluskey M, Williams H, Ogden GR. Vascularity and expression of vascular endothelial growth factor in oral squamous cell carcinoma, resection margins, and nodal metastases. *Br J Oral Maxillofac Surg.* 8: 2005.

In: Squamous Cell Carcinoma   ISBN: 978-1-61209-929-3
Editor: Daniel V. Mortensen   © 2012 Nova Science Publishers, Inc.

Chapter 12

LARYNGEAL SQUAMOUS CELL CARCINOMA: TREATMENT OPTIONS AND OUTCOMES

William M. Mendenhall[*1], *Russell W. Hinerman*[1], *Robert J. Amdur*[1], *Mikhail Vaysberg*[2] *and John W. Werning*[2]

[1]Department of Radiation Oncology, Health Science Center, University of Florida College of Medicine, Gainesville, FL, U.S.
[2]Department of Otolaryngology, University of Florida College of Medicine, Gainesville, FL, U.S.

ABSTRACT

The treatment alternatives for squamous cell carcinoma of the glottic and supraglottic larynx are discussed. The optimal treatment depends on the location and extent of the primary tumor, presence and extent of clinically postive nodes, and the medical condition of the patient.

[*] Corresponding author: Department of Radiation Oncology, University of Florida Health Science Center, P.O. Box 100385, Gainesville, FL 32610-0385, (Street address: 2000 SW Archer Road, 32608), Telephone: (352) 265-0287 Fax: (352) 265-0759, E-mail: mendwm@shands.ufl.edu

Treatment selection is addressed and the outcomes after radiotherapy and/or surgery are presented.

ANATOMY

The larynx is divided into the supraglottis, glottis, and subglottis. The supraglottis consists of the epiglottis, false vocal cords, ventricles, aryepiglottic folds, and the arytenoids. The glottis includes the true vocal cords and the anterior commissure. The lateral line of demarcation between the glottis and supraglottis is the apex of the ventricle. The subglottis is located below the vocal cords and is considered to extend from a point 5 mm below the free margin of the vocal cord to the inferior aspect of the cricoid cartilage.

The supraglottis has a rich capillary lymphatic plexus; the trunks pass through the preepiglottic space and the thyrohyoid membrane and terminate mainly in the level II lymph nodes; a few drain to the level III lymph nodes. There are essentially no capillary lymphatics of the true vocal cords, so that lymphatic spread occurs only if tumor extends to supraglottis or subglottis. The subglottis has relatively few capillary lymphatics. The lymphatic trunks pass through the cricothyroid membrane to the pretracheal (Delphian) lymph nodes in the region of the thyroid isthmus. The subglottis also drains posteriorly through the cricotracheal membrane, with some trunks going to the paratracheal lymph nodes (level VI) and others continuing to the inferior jugular chain (level IV).

DIAGNOSTIC EVALUATION

The diagnostic evaluation includes a physical examination (including flexible laryngoscopy), chest radiography, computed tomography (CT) of the larynx and neck, and direct laryngoscopy and biopsy. Nearly all malignant tumors of the larynx arise from the surface epithelium and are squamous cell carcinoma or one of its variants. Position emission tomography (PET) and magnetic resonance imaging (MRI) are obtained only to clarify an equivocal finding on CT or chest radiography.

STAGING

The 2002 American Joint Committee on Cancer (AJCC)[1] staging system for laryngeal primary cancer is listed in Table 1. T2 glottic cancers are stratified into those with normal (T2A) and impaired (T2B) vocal cord mobility. The major difference between the 1998 and 2002 staging systems is that a glottic cancer that invades the paraglottic space is upstaged to T3 in the latter system, even with mobile vocal cords, resulting in significant stage migration.

**Table 1. 2002 American Joint Committee on
Cancer (AJCC) Staging of laryngeal cancer**

Supraglottis	
T1	Tumor limited to one subsite of supraglottis with normal vocal cord mobility
T2	Tumor invades mucosa of more than one adjacent subsite of supraglottis or glottis or region outside the supraglottis (e.g., mucosa of base of tongue, vallecula, medial wall of pyriform sinus) without fixation of the larynx
T3	Tumor limited to larynx with vocal cord fixation and/or invades any of the following: postcricoid area, preepiglottic tissues, paraglottic space, and/or minor thyroid erosion (e.g., inner cortex)
T4a	Tumor invades through the thyroid cartilage and/or invades beyond the larynx (e.g., trachea, soft tissues of neck including deep extrinsic muscle of the tongue, strap muscles, thyroid, or esophagus)
T4b	Tumor invades prevertebral space, encases carotid artery, or invades mediastinal structures
Glottis	
T1	Tumor limited to vocal cord(s) (may involve anterior or posterior commissure) with normal mobility
T1a	Tumor limited to one vocal cord
T1b	Tumor involves both vocal cords
T2	Tumor extends to supraglottis and/or subglottis, and/or with impaired vocal cord mobility
T3	Tumor limited to the larynx with vocal cord fixation and/or invades paraglottic space, and/or minor thyroid cartilage erosion (e.g., inner cortex)
T4a	Tumor invades through the thyroid cartilage and/or invades tissues beyond the larynx (trachea, soft tissues of neck including deep extrinsic muscle of the tongue, strap muscles, thyroid, or esophagus}
T4b	Tumor invades prevertebral space, encases carotid artery, or invades mediastinal structures

(Modified from American Joint Committee on Cancer: Manual for Staging of Cancer, ed 6, pp. 47–57, New York: Springer-Verlag, 2002)[1]

TREATMENT SELECTION FOR GLOTTIC CARCINOMA

We have not adopted this latter modification and stage glottic cancers as T3 only if cord mobility is absent. Additionally, T4 has been stratified into T4A and T4B, based on resectability.

The goals of treatment include cure with the best functional result and the least risk of a serious complication. Patients are considered to be in an early group if the chance of cure with larynx preservation is high, a moderately advanced group if the likelihood of local control is 60% to 70% but the chance of cure remains good, and an advanced group if the chance of cure is moderate and the likelihood of laryngeal preservation is relatively low. The early group may be treated initially by radiation therapy (RT) or, in selected cases, by partial laryngectomy. The moderately advanced group may be treated with either RT with laryngectomy reserved for relapse or by total laryngectomy with or without adjuvant postoperative RT. A modest subset of these patients is suitable for an open partial laryngectomy (OPL). The obvious advantage of definitive RT or OPL, which we prefer at the University of Florida, is that there is a fairly good chance that the larynx will be preserved. Although some patients may be rehabilitated with a tracheoesophageal puncture (TEP) after total laryngectomy, only about 20% of patients use this device long term and the majority use an electric larynx.[2] The advanced group is treated with total laryngectomy and neck dissection with or without adjuvant RT or RT and adjuvant chemotherapy.[3] Recent data indicates that, whereas induction chemotherapy probably does not improve the likelihood of local-regional control and survival, concomitant chemotherapy and RT results in an improved possibility of cure compared with RT alone.[3-5] There is a subset of patients with high volume, unfavorable, advanced cancers who may be cured by chemoradiation but have a non-functional larynx and permanent tracheostomy and/or gastrostomy.[6] These patients are best treated with a total laryngectomy, neck dissection, and postoperative RT.

Early Glottic Carcinoma

In most centers, RT is the initial treatment for T1-T2N0 cancers, with surgery reserved for salvage.[7,8] The likelihood of lymph node metastases is low so the RT portals include only the primary site with a margin.[9] Patients are treated at 2.25 Gy per once daily fraction to 63 Gy for T_1-T_{2A} cancers and

65.25 Gy for T_{2B} tumors.[7,10 8,11] Patients with early lesions, particularly those limited to the mid-third of one cord, have a high likelihood of cure with good voice quality after transoral laser. [8,12,13] OPL also provides a high likelihood of cure in selected patients, but at the cost of poorer voice quality. [8] Supracricoid laryngectomy, as reported by Laccourreye et al.,[14] is a procedure designed to remove moderate-sized cancers involving the supraglottic and glottic larynx. The larynx may be removed with preservation of the cricoid and the arytenoid with its neurovascular innervation, the defect is closed by approximating the base of the tongue to the remaining larynx. The oncologic and functional results of this procedure in selected patients are reported to be excellent. OPL finds its major use as salvage surgery in suitable cases after RT failure.

Moderately Advanced Glottic Carcinoma

Fixed-cord lesions (T3) are stratified into relatively favorable or unfavorable subsets. Patients with unfavorable lesions usually have extensive bilateral disease with a compromised airway. Patients with favorable T3 lesions have disease confined mostly to one side of the larynx, have a good airway, and are reliable for follow-up. Some degree of supraglottic and subglottic extension usually exists. The extent of disease and tumor volume, in particular, are related to the likelihood of control after definitive RT.[6]

The patient with a favorable lesion is treated with RT or an OPL.[15,16] Recent data suggest that the likelihood of local–regional control is better after some altered fractionation schedules compared with conventional once-daily RT. We prefer 74.4 in 62 twice-daily fractions if the patient is treated with conventional RT, and 72 Gy in 42 fractions over 6 weeks using the concomitant boost technique if the patient is treated with intensity modulated radiation therapy (IMRT).[3,17] Additionally, concomitant chemotherapy and RT has been shown to improve the likelihood of cure compared with RT alone.[4] The optimal chemotherapy regimen is unclear.[4,5] The risk of subclinical regional disease is 20% to 30% so that the clinically negative neck is electively irradiated. Follow-up examinations are recommended every 4 to 6 weeks for the first year, every 2 months for the second year, every 3 months for the third year, every 6 months for the fourth and fifth years, and annually thereafter.

Advanced Glottic Carcinoma

Advanced lesions usually show extensive subglottic and supraglottic extension, bilateral glottic involvement, and invasion of the thyroid, cricoid, and/or arytenoid cartilages.[18,19] The airway is compromised, necessitating a tracheostomy at the time of direct laryngoscopy in approximately 30% of patients. Clinically positive lymph nodes are found in about 25% to 30% of patients.

Patients with unfavorable lesions are less likely to be cured with chemoradiation and more likely to have a functionless larynx if the tumor is eradicated. Thus, the majority of these patients are best treated with a total laryngectomy and neck dissection, with or without adjuvant RT. The indications for postoperative RT include close or positive margins, subglottic extension ($\geq$ 1 cm), cartilage invasion, perineural invasion, endothelial-lined space invasion, extension of the primary tumor into the soft tissues of the neck, multiple positive neck nodes, extracapsular extension, and control of subclinical disease in the opposite neck.[20,21] In practice, the vast majority of patients receive postoperative RT. Concomitant chemotherapy is given with postoperative RT for patients with positive margins and/or extracapsular extension. The postoperative RT dose is: negative margins, 60 Gy in 30 fractions; microscopic positive margins, 66 Gy in 33 fractions; and gross residual, 70 Gy in 35 fractions. The low neck received 50 Gy in 25 fractions; the stoma is boosted to 60 Gy with electrons if there is subglottic extension. IMRT may be employed to avoid a difficult low neck match. This is unnecessary in most patients. Preoperative RT is indicated for patients who have fixed neck nodes, have had an emergency tracheotomy through tumor, or have direct extension of tumor involving the skin.

TREATMENT SELECTION FOR
SUPRAGLOTTIC CARCINOMA

Early and Moderately Advanced Supraglottic Carcinoma

Treatment of the primary lesion for the early group is by RT or supraglottic laryngectomy, with or without adjuvant RT.[22] Approximately 50% of supraglottic laryngectomies performed at the University of Florida have been followed by postoperative RT because of neck disease and, less often, positive margins. Transoral laser excision is effective in experienced hands for small, selected lesions.[13] Total laryngectomy is reserved for treatment failures.

The decision to use RT or supraglottic laryngectomy depends on the anatomic extent of the tumor, medical condition of the patient, philosophy of the attending physician(s), and the inclination of the patient and family. Extension of the tumor to the true vocal cord, anterior commissure, vocal cord fixation, and/or thyroid or cricoid cartilage invasion precludes supraglottic laryngectomy. The procedure may be extended to include the base of tongue if one lingual artery is preserved. Supracricoid laryngectomy is an option for lesions involving one or both vocal cords; at least one arytenoid must be preserved. Vocal cord fixation and/or cartilage destruction are relative contraindications to this procedure. Overall, about 80% of patients are treated initially by RT. Approximately half of the patients seen in our clinic whose lesions are technically suitable for a supraglottic laryngectomy are not operable for medical reasons (e.g., inadequate pulmonary status or other major medical problems).

Analysis of local control by anatomic site within the supraglottic larynx shows no obvious differences in local control by RT for similarly staged lesions. Primary tumor volume based on pretreatment CT is inversely related to local tumor control after RT.[6] A large, bulky infiltrative lesion is a common reason to select supraglottic laryngectomy, as local control is probably improved compared to treatment with RT alone.

The status of the neck often determines the selection of treatment of the primary lesion. Patients with clinically negative neck nodes have a high risk for occult neck disease and may be treated by RT or supraglottic laryngectomy and bilateral selective neck dissections, (levels II-IV).

If a patient has an early-stage primary lesion and N2b or N3 neck disease, combined treatment is frequently necessary to control the neck disease.[23] In these cases, the primary lesion is usually treated by RT and concomitant chemotherapy. CT is obtained 4 weeks after RT and neck dissection is added if the risk of residual cancer in the neck is thought to exceed 5%; otherwise the patient is observed and a CT is repeated in 3 months.[23] If the same patient were treated with supraglottic laryngectomy, neck dissection, and postoperative RT, the portals would unnecessarily include the primary site as well as the neck. If the patient has early, resectable neck disease (N1 or N2a) and surgery is elected for the primary site, postoperative RT is added only because of unexpected findings (e.g., positive margins, multiple positive nodes, extensive perineural invasion, or extracapsular extension). Positive margins should be unusual after supraglottic laryngectomy if patients are selected appropriately. The primary site and neck are treated to 55.8 Gy at 1.8 Gy per fraction; the involved neck is boosted to 60 Gy to 70 Gy depending on the risk of residual disease.

Advanced Supraglottic Carcinoma

Although a subset of these patients may be suitable for a supraglottic or supracricoid laryngectomy, total laryngectomy is the main surgical option. Selected advanced lesions, especially those that are mainly exophytic, may be treated by RT and concomitant chemotherapy[5] with total laryngectomy reserved for RT failures. As is the case with the glottic larynx, patients cured by RT are more likely to have a functionless larynx.

For patients whose primary lesion is to be treated by a total or partial laryngectomy and who have resectable neck disease, surgery is the initial treatment, and postoperative RT is added if needed. If the neck disease is unresectable, preoperative RT is used. The indications for preoperative and postoperative RT have been previously outlined.

RESULTS OF TREATMENT

Glottic Carcinoma

The local control rates after treatment of early-stage glottic carcinoma are depicted in Tables 2 through 4.[8] The local control rates are similar for transoral laser excision, OPL, and RT. Larynx preservation and survival rates are also comparable. Voice quality depends on the amount of tissue removed with partial laryngectomy and is probably similar for patients with limited lesions treated with laser to those undergoing RT and poorer for patients undergoing an OPL.[8]

Foote and coworkers[24] reported on 81 patients who underwent laryngectomy for T3 cancers at the Mayo Clinic between 1970 and 1981. Seventy-five patients underwent a total laryngectomy and six underwent a near-total laryngectomy; 53 patients received a neck dissection. No patient received adjuvant RT or chemotherapy. The 5-year rates of local-regional control, cause-specific survival, and absolute survival were 74%, 74%, and 54%, respectively. The results of definitive RT patients with T3 glottic carcinoma are depicted in Table 5[25] and are similar to the surgical outcomes reported by Foote et al.[24]

Table 2. Local Control after Transoral Laser Excision

Institution	Follow-up*	No. pts.	Stage	Local Control (interval)	Local Control with Larynx Preservation (interval)	Ultimate Local Control (interval)
University of Göttingen [13]	Median, 78 mo	159	pTis-pT2	94% (NS)	99% (NS)	——
University of Kiel [28]	Mean, 40 mo	8	pTis	100% (NS)	——	——
		88	pT1a	92% (NS)	——	——
		10	pT1b	80% (NS)	——	——
		8	pT2	88% (NS)	——	——
		114	pTis-pT2	——	96% (NS)	——
University of Brescia [29]	Mean, 76 mo	21	pTis	81% (NS)	—	95%† (5 y)
		96	pT1	82% (NS)	——	87%† (5 y)
		23	pT2	74% (NS)	——	91%† (5 y)
		140	pTis-pT2	80% (NS)	97% (NS)	
Washington University [30]	Minimum, 3 y	61	T1	77% (NS)	90% (NS)	98% (NS)
University of Naples [31]	Minimum, 5 y	321	T1	82%† (NS)	89%‡ (NS)	——
		158	T2	60%† (NS)	~ 67%‡ (NS)	——
La Sapienza University [32]	Minimum, 3 y	12	Tis	100% (NS)	100% (NS)	——
		120	T1a	94% (NS)	100% (NS)	——
		24	T1b	91% (NS)	100% (NS)	——
Tata Memorial Hospital [33]	Minimum, 18 mo	52	T1a	90% (NS)	94% (NS)	——
		17	T1b	65% (NS)	88% (NS)	——
		13	T2	77% (NS)	92% (NS)	——

*Follow-up period for total number of patients; †Ultimate local control with laser treatment alone; ‡ Local–regional control rate; NS = not stated; y = years;mo = months.
(Mendenhall WM, Werning JW, Hinerman RW, Amdur RJ, Villaret DB. Management of T1–T2 glottic carcinomas Cancer 2004;100:1786–1792)[8] [Table 1,p 1787]

Table 3. Local Control after Open Partial Laryngectomy

Institution	Follow-up	No. Pts.	Stage	Local Control (interval)	Local Control with Larynx Preservation (interval)	Ultimate Local Control (interval)
Universitaire Timone [34]	NS	62	T1	100% (NS)	100% (NS)	——
		65	T2	92% (NS)	92% (NS)	——
Hôpital Saint Charles [35]	Minimum, 3 y	18	T1a	100% (NS)	——	——
		40	T1b	95% (NS)	——	——
		23	T2a	83% (NS)	——	——
Mayo Clinic [36]	Median, 6.6 y	159	Tis–T1	93% (5 y)	94% (NS)	100% (NS)
Hôpital Laënnec [37]	Minimum, 3 y	295	T1	89% (NS)	——	——
		90	T2a	74% (NS)	——	——
		31	T2b	68% (NS)	——	——
		416	T1–T2b	84% (NS)	——	97% (NS)

NS = not stated; y = years
(Mendenhall WM, Werning JW, Hinerman RW, Amdur RJ, Villaret DB. Management of T1–T2 glottic carcinomas. Cancer 2004;100:1786–1792)[8] [Table 2,p 1788]

Table 4. Local Control after Radiotherapy

Institution	Follow-up*	No. pts.	Stage	Local Control nterval)	Local Control with Larynx Preservation (interval)	Ultimate Local Control (interval)
University of Florida [7]	Minimum, 2 y Median, 9.9 y	230 61 146 82	T1a T1b T2a T2b	94% (5 y) 93% (5 y) 80% (5 y) 72% (5 y)	95% (5 y) 95% (5 y) 82% (5 y) 76% (5 y)	98% (5 y) 98% (5 y) 96% (5 y) 96% (5 y)
Massachusetts General Hospital [39]	NS	665	T1	93% (5 y)	——	——
		145	T2a	77% (5 y)	——	——
		92	T2b	71% (5 y)	——	——
University of California (SF) [40]	Median, 9.7 y	315 83	T1 T2	85% (5 y) 70% (5 y)	—— ——	96%† (5 y) 91%† (5 y)
Princess Margaret Hospital [41]	Median, 6.8 y	403 46 286	T1a T1b T2	91% (5 y) 82% (5 y) 69% (5 y)	—— —— ——	—— —— ——
M. D. Anderson Hospital [42]	Median, 6.8 y	114 116 230	T2a T2b T2	74% (5 y) 70% (5 y) 72% (5 y)	—— —— ——	—— —— 91% (5 y)

*Follow-up period for total number of patients; NS = not stated; y = years.
†Local–regional control rates.
(Mendenhall WM, Werning JW, Hinerman RW, Amdur RJ, Villaret DB. Management of T1–T2
glottic carcinomas. Cancer 2004;100:1786–1792)[8] [Table 3,p 1789]

Table 5. Stage T3 glottic carcinoma treated with irradiation alone (no chemotherapy)

Investigator	Institution	No. pts.	Minimum follow-up (y)	Local control (%)	Ultimate control after salvage surgery (%)
Harwood et al [43]	Princess Margaret (Toronto)	112	3	51	77
Wang [44]	Mass. General (Boston)	70	4	36	57
Fletcher et al [45]	M.D. Anderson (Houston)	17	2	77	No data
Skolyszewski and Reinfuss [46]	15 European Centers	91	3	50	No data
Stewart et al [47]	Manchester (England)	67	10	57	67
Mills [48]	Capetown, South Africa.	18	2	44	78
Hinerman et al. [27]	U. Florida (Gainesville)	87	2	63	89

(Modified from Parsons JT, Mendenhall WM, Mancuso AA, Cassisi NJ, Stringer SP, Million RR.
Twice-a-day radiotherapy for T3 squamous cell carcinoma of the glottic larynx. Head Neck
11:123-128, 1989)[25] [Table 2, p 127]

Table 6. Treatment of stage T4 glottic carcinomas

Investigator	Tumor stage	No. pts.	Method of treatment	Results (NED)
Jesse [49]	T4N0-N+	48	Laryngectomy	54% at 4 yr
Ogura et al. [50]	T4N0	11	Laryngectomy	45% at 3 yr
Skolnick et al. [51]	T4N0	7	Laryngectomy	30% at 5 yr
Vermund [52]	T4N0	31	Laryngectomy	35% at 5 yr
Stewart and Jackson [53]	T4N0	13	Radiotherapy with surgery for salvage	38% at 5 yr
Harwood et al. [26]	T4N0	56	Radiotherapy with surgery for salvage	49% at 5 yr*
Hinerman et al. [27]	T4N0	22	Radiotherapy with surgery for salvage	81% local control at 5yr.*

NED = no evidence of disease; *Life-table method; uncorrected for deaths from intercurrent disease.

(Modified from Harwood AR, Beal FA, Cummings BJ, Keane TJ, Payne D, Rider WD. T4N0M0 glottic cancer: An analysis of dose-time-volume. Int J Radiat Oncol Biol Phys 1981;7:1507–1512)[26] [Table 4, p 1511]

Table 7. Supraglottic Larynx: Local control after transoral laser excision

Series	Staging	No. pts.	Percent of patients with T1 or T2 tumors	Local control			
				T1	T2	T3	T4
Davis et al., 1991 [54]	P	14 R	57	100%	100%	50%	—
Steiner, 1993* [13]	P	81 R	72	—	76%	77%	100%
Zeitels et al., 1994 [55]	ND	22	100	100%	100%	—	—
Zeitels et al., 1994 [55]	ND	23 R	65	100%	92%	63%	—
Csanády et al., 1999 [56]	ND	23	100	70%†		—	—
Rudert et al., 1999 [57]	P	34 R	50	100%	75%	78%	38%

*51 glottic and 30 supraglottic; †overall local control rates for T1 and T2; P = pathologic staging; R = plus or minus radiotherapy; ND = type of staging not provided.

Note: Some figures were estimated as closely as possible to fit table format if the information was not specifically stated in the cited reference.

(Hinerman RW, Mendenhall WM, Amdur RJ, Stringer SP, Villaret DB, Robbins KT. Carcinoma of the supraglottic larynx: Treatment results with radiotherapy alone or with planned neck dissection. Head Neck 24:456-467, 2002)[22] [Table 5, p 463]

Table 8. Supraglottic Larynx: Local control after radiotherapy

Series	Institution	No. pts.	T1	T2	T3	T4
Fletcher and Hamberger, 1974[58]	M.D. Anderson Hospital	173	88%	79%	62%	47%
Ghossein et al., 1974[59]	Fondation Curie	203	94%	73%	46%*	52%
Wang and Montgomery, 1991[60]	Massachusetts General Hospital	229 q.d. 209 b.i.d.	73% 89%	60% 89%	54% 71%	26% 91%
Nakfoor et al, 1998[61]	Massachusetts General Hospital	164	96%	86%	76%	43%
Sykes et al., 2000[62]	Christie Hospital	331†	92%‡	81%‡	67%‡	73%‡
Hinerman et al.[22]	University of Florida§	274	100%	86%	62%	62%

*All had cord fixation; †all N0; ‡after 17 were salvaged by total laryngectomies; §1998 AJCC staging; q.d., once a day; b.i.d., twice a day.

Note: Some figures were estimated as closely as possible to fit table format if the information was not specifically stated in the cited reference.

(Hinerman RW, Mendenhall WM, Amdur RJ, Stringer SP, Villaret DB, Robbins KT. Carcinoma of the supraglottic larynx: Treatment results with radiotherapy alone or with planned neck dissection. Head Neck 24:456-467,2002)[22] [Table 6, p 463]

Table 9. Local control after supraglottic laryngectomy

Series	Institution	No. Pts.	Patients with T1 and T2 tumors (%)	Local control T1 (%)	T2 (%)	T3 (%)	T4 (%)
Ogura et al, 1975[63]	Washington University	177	78	—	94*	—	—
Bocca, 1991[64]	Milan University						
Stage I		47	100	94	—	—	—
Stage II		252	100	—	82	—	—
Stage III		205	53	—	80†	—	—
Stage IV		33	70	—	67‡	—	—
Lee et al, 1990[65]	M.D. Anderson Cancer Center	60	58	100	100	100	100
DeSanto, 1990[66]	Mayo Clinic	70	100	100	100	—	—
Steiniger et al, 1997[67]	Albany Medical College	29	83	—	97*	—	—
Spriano et al, 1997[68]	Varese, Italy	54	100	96§	—	—	—
Burstein and Calcattera, 1985[69]	University of California (LA)	40	58	100		85	94
Isaacs et al, 1998[70]	University of Florida	33	76	100		78	71
Lutz et al, 1990[71]	University of Pittsburgh	72	No data	—	99¶	—	—

*Overall local control rates for T1–T4; †Overall local control rates for T1–T3; ‡Overall local control rates for T2–T3; §Overall local control rates for T1–T2;

T stages were not specified.

Note: Some figures were estimated as closely as possible to fit table format if the information was not specifically stated in the cited reference.

(Hinerman RW, Mendenhall WM, Amdur RJ, Stringer SP, Villaret DB, Robbins KT. Carcinoma of the supraglottic larynx: Treatment results with radiotherapy alone or with planned neck dissection. Head Neck 24:456, 2002)[22] [Table 7, p 464]

Table 10. Supraglottic Larynx: Severe complications
according to treatment modality

Series	Institution	No. of severe complications
	Radiotherapy	
Fletcher and Hamberger, 1974[58]	M.D. Anderson Cancer Center	10/173 (6%)
Ghossein et al., 1974[59]	Fondation Curie	8/117 (7%)
Nakfoor et al., 1998[61]	Massachusetts General Hospital	12/169 (7%)
Sykes et al., 2000[62]	Christie Hospital	7/331 (2%)
Hinerman et al.[22]	University of Florida	12/274 (4%)
	Supraglottic laryngectomy	
Lee et al., 1991[65]	M.D. Anderson Cancer Center	9/63 (14%)
Isaacs et al., 1998[70]	University of Florida	14/34 (41%)
Burstein and Calcaterra, 1985[69]	University of California Los Angeles	14/41 (34%)
Steiniger et al., 1997[67]	Albany Medical College	12/29 (41%)
Spriano et al., 1997[68]	Varese, Italy	13/54 (24%)
Gall et al., 1977[72]	Washington University	20/133 (15%)
Weber et al., 1993[73]	University of Pittsburgh	12/69 (17%)
Beckhardt et al., 1994[74]	University of Wisconsin	15/50 (30%)
	Transoral laser excision	
Rudert et al., 1999[57]	University of Kiel, Germany	3/34 (9%)
Zeitels et al., 1994[55]	Massachusetts Eye and Ear Infirmary	2/45 (4%)
Steiner, 1993*[13]	University of Gottingen, Germany	7/240 (3%)
Davis et al., 1991[54]	University of Utah, Salt Lake City	0/14 (0%)
Csanády et al., 1999[56]	Albert Szent Gyorgyi Medical University, Szeged, Hungary	0/23 (0%)

*Includes patients with glottic cancer.
Note: Some figures were estimated as closely as possible to fit table format if the information was not specifically stated in the cited reference.
(Hinerman RW, Mendenhall WM, Amdur RJ, Stringer SP, Villaret DB, Robbins KT. Carcinoma of the supraglottic larynx: Treatment results with radiotherapy alone or with planned neck dissection. Head Neck 24:456-467, 2002)[22] [Table 8, p 465]

The 5-year outcomes after RT (53 patients) versus surgery with or without RT (65 patients) for patients with T3 fixed-cord lesions treated at the University of Florida were: local-regional control, 62% vs. 75%; ultimate local-regional control, 84% vs. 82%; absolute survival, 55% vs. 45%; and cause-specific survival, 75% vs. 71%.[19] There was no relationship between subsequent local control and whether the vocal cord remained fixed or became mobile during RT. The incidence of severe complications, including those after the initial treatment and any later salvage procedures, was 15% after RT alone and 15% after surgery alone or combined with adjuvant RT. Vocal quality varied from fair to nearly normal.

The results of treatment of T4 vocal cord carcinoma in four surgical series and three RT series are summarized in Table 6.[26] Hinerman et al reported on 22 highly selected patients with low volume T_4 cancers treated with definitive RT; the 5-year local control rate was 81%.[27]

Supraglottic Carcinoma

The proportion of patients suitable for a supraglottic laryngectomy is variable.[22] Depending on the referral patterns, a modest subset of patients is suitable for this operation. The extent of neck disease in patients treated with either surgery or radiotherapy is also variable.[22] In general, patients treated with supraglottic laryngectomy appropriately have earlier stage neck disease and would be anticipated to have a lower risk of distant failure and improved survival. The local control rates after transoral laser, RT, and supraglottic laryngectomy are summarized in Tables 7, 8, and 9.[22] In general, the local control rates after transoral laser excision are fairly good for patients with T1–T2 tumors and tend to deteriorate for those with more advanced disease. The local control rate for patients selected for supraglottic laryngectomy are excellent. However, the incidence of severe complications tends to be higher after supraglottic laryngectomy compared with RT and transoral laser excision (Table 10).[22]

CONCLUSIONS

Patients with early laryngeal carcinomas have a high chance of cure after RT or partial laryngectomy. Those with moderately advanced carcinomas are optimally treated with RT and concomitant chemotherapy or partial laryngectomy alone or combined with adjuvant RT. Patients with advanced carcinomas after require a total laryngectomy and neck dissection followed by postoperative RT.

ACKNOWLEDGMENT

We thank the research support staff of the Department of Radiation Oncology for their help with statistics, editing, and manuscript preparation.

REFERENCES

[1]   American Joint Committee on Cancer. Larynx. *AJCC Cancer Staging Manual*, ed. 6. New York: Springer, 2002, 47-57.

[2]   Mendenhall, WM; Morris, CG; Stringer, SP; et al. Voice rehabilitation after total laryngectomy and postoperative radiation therapy. *J Clin Oncol.*, 2002, 20, 2500-2505.

[3]   Mendenhall, WM; Riggs, CE; Amdur, RJ; et al. Altered fractionation and/or adjuvant chemotherapy in definitive irradiation of squamous cell carcinoma of the head and neck. *Laryngoscope*, 2003, 113, 546-551.

[4]   Forastiere, AA; Goepfert, H; Maor, M; et al. Concurrent chemotherapy and radiotherapy for organ preservation in advanced laryngeal cancer. *N Engl J Med.*, 2003, 349, 2091-2098.

[5]   Pignon, JP; Bourhis, J; Domenge, C; et al. Chemotherapy added to locoregional treatment for head and neck squamous-cell carcinoma: Three meta-analyses of updated individual data. *Lancet*, 2000, 355, 949-955.

[6]   Mendenhall, WM; Morris, CG; Amdur, RJ; et al. Parameters that predict local control following definitive radiotherapy for squamous cell carcinoma of the head and neck. *Head Neck*, 2003, 25, 535-542.

[7]   Mendenhall, WM; Amdur, RJ; Morris, CG; et al. T1-T2N0 squamous cell carcinoma of the glottic larynx treated with radiation therapy. *J Clin Oncol.*, 2001, 19, 4029-4036.

[8]   Mendenhall, WM; Werning, JW; Hinerman, RW; et al. Management of T1-T2 glottic carcinomas. *Cancer*, 2004, 100, 1786-1792.

[9]   Million, RR; Cassisi, NJ; Mancuso, AA. Larynx. In: R. R. Million, & N. J. Cassisi, (Eds.), *Management of Head and Neck Cancer: A Multidisciplinary Approach*, ed. 2. Philadelphia: J. B. Lippincott Company, 1994, 431-497.

[10] Yamazaki, H; Nishiyama, K; Tanaka, E; et al. Radiotherapy for early glottic carcinoma (T1N0M0): Results of prospective randomized study of radiation fraction size and overall treatment time. *Int J Radiat Oncol Biol Phys.*, 2006, 64, 77-82.

[11] O'Sullivan, B; Mackillop, W; Gilbert, R; et al. Controversies in the management of laryngeal cancer: Results of an international survey of patterns of care. *Radiother Oncol.*, 1994, 31, 23-32.

[12] McGuirt, WF; Blalock, D; Koufman, JA; et al. Comparative voice results after laser resection or irradiation of T1 vocal cord carcinoma. *Arch Otolaryngol Head Neck Surg.*, 1994, 120, 951-955.

[13] Steiner, W. Results of curative laser microsurgery of laryngeal carcinomas. *Am J Otolaryngol.*, 1993, 14, 116-121.

[14] Laccourreye, H; Laccourreye, O; Weinstein, G; et al. Supracricoid laryngectomy with cricohyoidoepiglottopexy: A partial laryngeal procedure for glottic carcinoma. *Ann Otol Rhinol Laryngol.*, 1990, 99, 421-426.

[15] Hinni, ML; Salassa, JR; Grant, DG; et al. Transoral laser microsurgery for advanced laryngeal cancer. *Arch Otolaryngol Head Neck Surg.*, 2007, 133, 1198-1204.

[16] Lima, RA; Freitas, EQ; Dias, FL; et al. Supracricoid laryngectomy with cricohyoidoepiglottopexy for advanced glottic cancer. *Head Neck*, 2006, 28, 481-486.

[17] Fu, KK; Pajak, TF; Trotti, A; et al. A Radiation Therapy Oncology Group (RTOG) phase III randomized study to compare hyperfractionation and two variants of accelerated fractionation to standard fractionation radiotherapy for head and neck squamous cell carcinomas: First report of RTOG 9003. *Int J Radiat Oncol Biol Phys.*, 2000, 48, 7-16.

[18] Archer, CR; Yeager, VL; Herbold, DR. Improved diagnostic accuracy in laryngeal cancer using a new classification based on computed tomography. *Cancer*, 1984, 53, 44-57.

[19] Mendenhall, WM; Parsons, JT; Stringer, SP; et al. Stage T3 squamous cell carcinoma of the glottic larynx: A comparison of laryngectomy and irradiation. *Int J Radiat Oncol Biol Phys.*, 1992, 23, 725-732.

[20] Amdur, RJ; Parsons, JT; Mendenhall, WM; et al. Postoperative irradiation for squamous cell carcinoma of the head and neck: an analysis of treatment results and complications. *Int J Radiat Oncol Biol Phys.*, 1989, 16, 25-36.

[21] Huang, DT; Johnson, CR; Schmidt-Ullrich, R; et al. Postoperative radiotherapy in head and neck carcinoma with extracapsular lymph node extension and/or positive resection margins: a comparative study. *Int J Radiat Oncol Biol Phys.*, 1992, 23, 737-742.

[22] Hinerman, RW; Mendenhall, WM; Amdur, RJ; et al. Carcinoma of the supraglottic larynx: Treatment results with radiotherapy alone or with planned neck dissection. *Head Neck*, 2002, 24, 456-467.

[23] Mendenhall, WM; Villaret, DB; Amdur, RJ; et al. Planned neck dissection after definitive radiotherapy for squamous cell carcinoma of the head and neck. *Head Neck*, 2002, 24, 1012-1018.

[24] Foote, RL; Olsen, KD; Buskirk, SJ; et al. Laryngectomy alone for T3 glottic cancer. *Head Neck*, 1994, 16, 406-412.

[25] Parsons, JT; Mendenhall, WM; Mancuso, AA; et al. Twice-a-day radiotherapy for T3 squamous cell carcinoma of the glottic larynx. *Head Neck*, 1989, 11, 123-128.

[26] Harwood, AR; Beale, FA; Cummings, BJ; et al. T4N0M0 glottic cancer: An analysis of dose-time-volume factors. *Int J Radiat Oncol Biol Phys.*, 1981, 7, 1507-1512.

[27] Hinerman, RW; Mendenhall, WM; Morris, CG; et al. T3 and T4 true vocal cord squamous carcinomas treated with external beam irradiation: a single institution's 35-year experience. *Am J Clin Oncol.*, 2007, 30, 181-185.

[28] Rudert, HH; Werner, JA. Endoscopic resections of glottic and supraglottic carcinomas with the CO2 laser. *Eur Arch Otorhinolaryngol.*, 1995, 252, 146-148.

[29] Peretti, G; Nicolai, P; Redaelli De Zinis, LO; et al. Endoscopic CO2 laser excision for Tis, T1, and T2 glottic carcinomas: Cure rate and prognostic factors. *Otolaryngol Head Neck Surg.*, 2000, 123, 124-131.

[30] Spector, JG; Sessions, DG; Chao, KS; et al. Stage I (T1 N0 M0) squamous cell carcinoma of the laryngeal glottis: Therapeutic results and voice preservation. *Head Neck*, 1999, 21, 707-717.

[31] Motta, G; Esposito, E; Cassiano, B; et al. T1-T2-T3 glottic tumors: Fifteen years experience with CO_2 laser. *Acta Otolaryngol Suppl.*, 1997, 527, 155-159.

[32] Gallo, A; de Vincentiis, M; Manciocco, V; et al. CO2 laser cordectomy for early-stage glottic carcinoma: A long-term follow-up of 156 cases. *Laryngoscope*, 2003, 112,370-374.

[33] Pradhan, SA; Pai, PS; Neeli, SI; et al. Transoral laser surgery for early glottic cancers. *Arch Otolaryngol Head Neck Surg.*, 2003, 129, 623-625.

[34] Giovanni, A; Guelfucci, B; Gras, R; et al. Partial frontolateral laryngectomy with epiglottic reconstruction for management of early-stage glottic carcinoma. *Laryngoscope*, 2001, 111, 663-668.

[35] Crampette, L; Garrel, R; Gardiner, Q; et al. Modified subtotal laryngectomy with cricohyoidoepiglottopexy--Long term results in 81 patients. *Head Neck*, 1999, 21, 95-103.

[36] Thomas, JV; Olsen, KD; Neel, HB; III et al. Early glottic carcinoma treated with open laryngeal procedures. *Arch Otolaryngol Head Neck Surg.*, 1994, 120, 264-268.

[37] Laccourreye, O; Weinstein, G; Brasnu, D; et al. A clinical trial of continuous cisplatin-fluorouracil induction chemotherapy and supracricoid partial laryngectomy for glottic carcinoma classified as T2. *Cancer*, 1994, 74, 2781-2790.

[38] Spector, JG; Sessions, DG; Chao, KSC; et al. Management of stage II (T2N0M0) glottic carcinoma by radiotherapy and conservation surgery. *Head Neck*, 1999, 21, 116-123.

[39] Wang, CC. Carcinoma of the larynx. In: C. C. Wang, editor. *Radiation Therapy for Head and Neck Neoplasms*, ed. 3rd. New York: Wiley-Liss, Inc., 1997, 221-255.

[40] Le, QT; Fu, KK; Kroll, S; et al. Influence of fraction size, total dose, and overall time on local control of T1-T2 glottic carcinoma. *Int J Radiat Oncol Biol Phys.*, 1997, 39, 115-126.

[41] Warde, P; O'Sullivan, B; Bristow, RG; et al. T1-T2 glottic cancer managed by external beam radiotherapy: The influence of pretreatment hemoglobin on local control. *Int J Radiat Oncol Biol Phys.*, 1998, 41, 347-353.

[42] Garden, AS; Forster, K; Wong, PF; et al. Results of radiotherapy for T2N0 glottic carcinoma: Does the "2" stand for twice-daily treatment? *Int J Radiat Oncol Biol Phys.*, 2003, 55, 322-328.

[43] Harwood, AR; Beale, FA; Cummings, BJ; et al. T3 glottic cancer: An analysis of dose-time-volume factors. *Int J Radiat Oncol Biol Phys.*, 1980, 6, 675-680.

[44] Wang, CC. Radiation therapy of laryngeal tumors: Curative radiation therapy. In: S. E. Thawley, & W. R. Panje, (Eds.), *Comprehensive Management of Head and Neck Tumors*. Philadelphia: WB Saunders, 1987, 906-919.

[45] Fletcher, GH; Lindberg, RD; Jesse, RH. Radiation therapy for cancer of the larynx and pyriform sinus. *Eye Ear Nose Throat Digest*, 1969, 31, 58-67.

[46] Skolyszewski, J; Reinfuss, M. The results of radiotherapy of cancer of the larynx in six European countries. *Radiobiol Radiother (Berl)*, 1981, 22, 32-43.

[47] Stewart, JG; Brown, JR; Palmer, MK; et al. The management of glottic carcinoma by primary irradiation with surgery in reserve. *Laryngoscope*, 1975, 85, 1477-1484.

[48] Mills, EE. Early glottic carcinoma: Factors affecting radiation failure, results of treatment and sequelae. *Int J Radiat Oncol Biol Phys.*, 1979, 5, 811-817.

[49] Jesse, RH. The evaluation of treatment of patients with extensive squamous cancer of the vocal cords. *Laryngoscope*, 1975, 85, 1424-1429.

[50] Ogura, JH; Sessions, DG; Ciralsky, RH. Supraglottic carcinoma with extension to the arytenoid. *Laryngoscope*, 1975, 85, 1327-1331.

[51] Skolnik, EM; Yee, KF; Wheatley, MA; et al. Carcinoma of the laryngeal glottis: Therapy and end results. *Laryngoscope*, 1975, 85, 1453-1466.

[52] Vermund, H. Role of radiotherapy in cancer of the larynx as related to the TNM system of staging. A review. *Cancer*, 1970, 25, 485-504.

[53] Stewart, JG; Jackson, AW. The steepness of the dose response curve both for tumor cure and normal tissue injury. *Laryngoscope*, 1975, 85, 1107-1111.

[54] Davis, RK; Kelly, SM; Hayes, J. Endoscopic CO_2 laser excisional biopsy of early supraglottic cancer. *Laryngoscope*, 1991, 101, 680-683.

[55] Zeitels, SM; Koufman, JA; Davis, RK; et al. Endoscopic treatment of supraglottic and hypopharynx cancer. *Laryngoscope*, 1994, 104, 71-78.

[56] Csanády, M; Iván, L; Czigner, J. Endoscopic CO_2 laser therapy of selected cases of supraglottic marginal tumors. *Eur Arch Otorhinolaryngol.*, 1999, 256, 392-394.

[57] Rudert, HH; Werner, JA; Höft, S. Transoral carbon dioxide laser resection of supraglottic carcinoma. *Ann Otol Rhinol Laryngol.*, 1999, 108, 819-827.

[58] Fletcher, GH; Hamberger, AD. Causes of failure in irradiation of squamous-cell carcinoma of the supraglottic larynx. *Radiology*, 1974, 111, 697-700.

[59] Ghossein, NA; Bataini, JP; Ennuyer, A; et al. Local control and site of failure in radically irradiated supraglottic laryngeal cancer. *Radiology*, 1974, 112, 187-192.

[60] Wang, CC; Montgomery, WM. Deciding on optimal management of supraglottic carcinoma. *Oncology*, 1991, 5, 41-46.

[61] Nakfoor, BM; Spiro, IJ; Wang, CC; et al. Results of accelerated radiotherapy for supraglottic carcinoma: A Massachusetts General Hospital and Massachusetts Eye and Ear Infirmary experience. *Head Neck*, 1998, 20, 379-384.

[62] Sykes, AJ; Slevin, NJ; Gupta, NK; et al. 331 cases of clinically node-negative supraglottic carcinoma of the larynx: A study of a modest size

fixed field radiotherapy approach. *Int J Radiat Oncol Biol Phys.*, 2000, 46, 1109-1115.

[63] Ogura, JH; Sessions, DG; Spector, GJ. Conservation surgery for epidermoid carcinoma of the supraglottic larynx. *Laryngoscope*, 1975, 85, 1808-1815.

[64] Bocca, E; Sixteenth Daniel, C; Baker, Jr. Memorial Lecture. Surgical management of supraglottic cancer and its lymph node metastases in a conservative perspective. *Ann Otol Rhinol Laryngol.*, 1991, 100, 261-267.

[65] Lee, NK; Goepfert, H; Wendt, CD. Supraglottic laryngectomy for intermediate-stage cancer: U.T. M.D. Anderson Cancer Center experience with combined therapy. *Laryngoscope*, 1990, 100, 831-836.

[66] DeSanto, LW. Early supraglottic cancer. *Ann Otol Rhinol Laryngol.*, 1990, 99, 593-597.

[67] Steiniger, JR; Parnes, SM; Gardner, GM. Morbidity of combined therapy for the treatment of supraglottic carcinoma: Supraglottic laryngectomy and radiotherapy. *Ann Otol Rhinol Laryngol.*, 1997, 106, 151-158.

[68] Spriano, G; Antognoni, P; Piantanida, R; et al. Conservative management of T1-T2N0 supraglottic cancer: A retrospective study. *Am J Otolaryngol.*, 1997, 18, 299-305.

[69] Burstein, FD; Calcaterra, TC. Supraglottic laryngectomy: Series report and analysis of results. *Laryngoscope*, 1985, 95, 833-836.

[70] Isaacs, JH Jr; Slattery, WH III, Mendenhall, WM; et al. Supraglottic laryngectomy. *Am J Otolaryngol.*, 1998, 19, 118-123.

[71] Lutz, CK; Johnson, JT; Wagner, RL; et al. Supraglottic carcinoma: Patterns of recurrence. *Ann Otol Rhinol Laryngol.*, 1990, 99, 12-17.

[72] Gall, AM; Sessions, DG; Ogura, JH. Complications following surgery for cancer of the larynx and hypopharynx. *Cancer*, 1977, 39, 624-631.

[73] Weber, PC; Johnson, JT; Myers, EN. Impact of bilateral neck dissection on recovery following supraglottic laryngectomy. *Arch Otolaryngol Head Neck Surg.*, 1993, 119, 61-64.

[74] Beckhardt, RN; Murray, JG; Ford, CN; et al. Factors influencing functional outcome in supraglottic laryngectomy. *Head Neck*, 1994, 16, 232-239.

INDEX

A

ABC, 218
aberrant, 215, 226
abnormalities, 215
access, 208
accounting, 140
acetaldehyde, 73
acetic acid, 203
acetone, 218
acid, xi, xiii, 39, 126, 127, 129, 132, 133, 134, 135
acidic, 62
acquisitions, 173
acute lymphoblastic leukemia, 26, 36, 37
ADC, 20, 21, 41
adenocarcinoma, 20, 21, 41, 42, 46, 53, 67
adenomatous polyposis coli, 57, 64
adenopathy, 195
adhesion, 17, 32, 51, 55, 56, 57, 60, 63, 64, 66, 67, 68
advancement, 13
aerodigestive tract, 10, 83, 192, 196, 223
aetiology, 84, 85, 151
Africa, 84
age, 6, 63, 72, 73, 74, 84, 93, 102, 103, 110, 111, 114, 145, 150, 151, 219
aggressiveness, 112, 141
airway epithelial cells, 34

airways, 15, 19, 20, 22, 28, 40, 41, 42, 43, 45, 46
alcohol, 215, 219, 220, 224
alcohol abuse, 46
alcohol consumption, 73
alcohol use, 151, 219
algorithm, 160
allele, 7, 11, 42, 70
allelic loss, 41, 65
alternative, 224
alters, 60
alveolar ridge, 75
alveoli, 15, 19
amino, 55
amino acid, 55
amino acids, 55
amputation, 118, 120
anatomic site, 50, 235
anatomy, 157, 161, 166, 172
anchorage, 66
anchoring, 54, 56
anemia, 73
aneuploid, 209
angiogenesis, 26, 27, 35, 37, 196, 197, 227
angiogenic, 224
angiography, 193, 194
Antibodies, 218
antibody, 130, 192, 218, 219, 220, 227
anti-cancer, xiii, 126, 127, 128, 129, 132, 133, 134, 135

antigen, 4, 78, 87, 135, 224, 226
anus, xii, 92, 98
APC, 25, 46, 51, 52, 54, 55, 57, 58, 64, 66
apex, 230
apoptosis, xiii, 27, 49, 53, 66, 78, 80, 83, 89,
    126, 127, 129, 132, 133, 134, 135, 215,
    226
apoptosis pathways, 80
apoptotic, 225
apoptotic pathways, 126
arrest, 51, 78, 79, 215
arsenic, 151
arteries, 166, 191
artery, 171, 191, 194, 231, 235
Asia, 72
aspiration, 115
assault, 14
assessment, xiv, 29, 30, 142, 147, 156, 166,
    189, 190, 193, 209
asymptomatic, 24, 67, 74, 85, 203
attachment, 50
Australia, 226
autopsy, 77, 87
avoidance, 3

B

bacterial infection, 118
Bangladesh, 84
barriers, 141
basal cell carcinoma, 61, 67, 100, 101
basal layer, 17, 22, 54, 57, 62, 220
base, 76, 140, 141, 226, 231, 233, 235
basement membrane, 45, 49
benign, 60, 73, 85, 95, 101, 203, 226
benign tumors, 60
binding, 215
biological, 224
biomarkers, xv, 200, 202, 204, 205, 206,
    207, 208, 227
biomolecules, 202
biopsies, xvi, 214, 222, 223
biopsy, xv, 75, 114, 117, 123, 124, 186,
    200, 201, 202, 204, 207, 211, 230, 248
biotin, 218

bleeding, 75, 173
blood, 15, 19, 161, 166, 190, 191, 196
blood circulation, 166
blood flow, 191, 196
blood stream, 19
blood vessels, 15, 161
body fluid, 209
bone, 17, 76, 77, 152, 158, 165, 171, 182,
    186, 189
bone form, 17
bones, 157, 166
brain, xv, 11, 53, 200
brain cancer, 11
Brazil, 71, 82
breast cancer, 27, 33, 35
breast carcinoma, 35
breathing, 75
bronchial airways, 15
bronchial epithelial cells, 20, 41
bronchial epithelium, 10, 16, 28, 63, 70
bronchioles, 15, 19, 31
bronchus, 63
buccal mucosa, 50

C

Ca^{2+}, 66
cachexia, 75
calcification, 173
calcium, 56, 136
candidates, 3, 18
capillary, 192, 209, 230
capsule, 76
carbon, 248
carbon dioxide, 248
carboxyl, 55
carcinogen, 7, 8, 29, 79, 80, 81
carcinogenesis, x, 2, 4, 6, 8, 9, 10, 11, 13,
    19, 23, 29, 33, 34, 40, 41, 47, 48, 52, 54,
    62, 65, 70, 72, 79, 83, 88, 89, 110, 112,
    113, 122, 215
carcinogenic, 215
carcinogens, 215
cartilage, 15, 96, 165, 231, 234, 235
caspases, 80

causation, 7
cDNA, 66, 204
cervical cancer, 102, 107
cervical dysplasia, 102
cervix, ix, 1
challenges, 215
chemokine receptor, 33
chemokines, 3
chemoprevention, 117
chemotherapy, 78, 87, 120, 121, 126, 141,
    152, 192, 232, 233, 234, 235, 236, 239,
    243, 244
chest radiography, 230
children, 6
chromosomal abnormalities, 202
chromosomal instability, 211
chromosome, 5, 6, 61, 64, 70, 78, 89, 215
chronic irritation, 74
cigarette smoke, 10, 67
cigarette smokers, 67
cigarette smoking, 28, 226
City, 134, 242
classification, 34, 43, 76, 86, 111, 245
claustrophobia, 182
cleavage, 132, 133, 134, 135
clinical, 216, 219, 223
clinical application, 194
clinical diagnosis, xv, 75, 200
clinical presentation, 150, 151
clone, 12
cloning, 106
clustering, 65
clusters, 11
coal, 32
coal tar, 32
coding, 51
collaboration, 31
collagen, 49, 113, 123
colon, 9, 25, 32, 80
colon cancer, 9, 32
color, 24, 49
colorectal cancer, 34, 120
combined effect, 73
commercial, 207
commissure, 230, 231, 235

communication, 7
complement, 204
compliance, 115
complications, 242, 243, 245
composition, 15
compounds, 8
computed tomography, 156, 195, 196, 230,
    245
condensation, 126
congestive heart failure, 172
connective tissue, 49, 77
consensus, 120
conservation, 30, 247
constituents, 73
consumption, 151
contour, 180
contradiction, 133
control, 225, 226
control group, 81
controversial, 74
controversies, 84
correlation, xiv, 76, 84, 142, 145, 155, 192,
    216, 219, 220, 224
cortex, 231
cost, 183, 208, 233
counterbalance, 6
covering, 191, 201
cricoid cartilage, 230, 235
cricothyroid membrane, 230
crown, 36
CSCs, ix, 1, 12, 13, 14, 18, 19, 24
CT scan, xiii, 98, 118, 140, 172, 189
cues, x, 2, 47
cultivation, 30
cure, 232, 233, 243, 248
cyclin D1, 227
cycling, 78
cyclins, 79
cyst, xii, 91, 92, 93, 94, 95, 96, 97, 98, 100,
    101, 102, 103, 104, 105, 106, 107
cysteine, 26
cysts, 225
cytokines, 5, 17, 211
cytologic, 225
cytology, 67, 210

cytometry, 12
cytoplasm, 25, 43, 44, 49, 50, 51, 52, 54, 58,
    133, 134, 136, 180, 183
cytoskeleton, 54, 56, 210
cytotoxic agents, 79
cytotoxicity, 127, 134

D

database, 150, 205
death, 214
deaths, 72, 239
deconvolution, 196
defects, 25, 46, 80, 126
deficiency, 73
degradation, 25, 46, 51, 52, 69
Delta, 26
Denmark, 82
dephosphorylation, 127
depth, 77
deregulation, x, 2
dermatologist, 117
dermis, 95, 100, 102
desmosome, 56
desorption, 206
destruction, 51, 102, 235
detectable, 46, 81, 113, 133
detection, xii, xiii, xiv, xv, 12, 67, 72, 87,
    107, 114, 115, 118, 121, 133, 140, 142,
    156, 157, 158, 160, 166, 182, 185, 192,
    200, 202, 203, 204, 206, 209, 210, 226
developed countries, 46
diabetes, 172
diagnostic criteria, 20, 93
diagnostic markers, 205
diet, 73
dietary, 224
differential diagnosis, 67, 189
differentiation, 215, 227
diffusivity, 180, 182
discomfort, xv, 200
discontinuity, 158
disease progression, 70
diseases, xii, xiii, 11, 26, 73, 91, 101, 140,
    173

disorder, 13
dispersion, 191
displacement, 57, 171
distortions, 142
distribution, 3, 34, 36, 67, 72, 80, 107, 178,
    191, 192
dosage, 117, 120
drainage, 141
dressings, 114, 115
drinking, 215, 224
drug resistance, 3
drugs, xiii, 79, 126, 127, 129, 132, 133, 135
DWI, 180, 182
dysphagia, 75
dysplasia, 9, 20, 41, 43, 46, 49, 74, 77, 78,
    79, 89, 215, 222

E

E-cadherin, 51, 54, 55, 56, 57, 60, 63, 64,
    65, 66, 67, 68
edema, 179, 189
Egypt, 213, 216
electromagnetic, 172
electron, 63
electrons, 234
electrophoresis, 132, 205, 206, 212
ELISA, 206
emboli, 76
embolization, 76
embryogenesis, 25
emergency, 234
emission, 196, 230
enamel, 17
encoding, 26, 56
endocrine, 20, 41
endonuclease, 133
endothelial cells, 27, 37
energy, 157, 172, 183
England, 218, 239
enlargement, 75
environment, 3, 18, 30, 33, 60, 178, 191
environmental factors, 22, 89
equipment, 156, 157, 171
erosion, 171, 231

esophagus, ix, 231
estrogen, 35
etiology, 73
Europe, 195
European Union, 72
evidence, xv, 10, 11, 12, 13, 20, 23, 29, 51, 70, 83, 87, 106, 113, 118, 120, 136, 192, 207, 214, 215, 216, 239
evolution, 19, 32, 40, 157, 210
examinations, 77, 145, 233
excision, xiii, 115, 118, 121, 147, 152, 216, 234, 236, 240, 242, 243, 246
execution, 4
exfoliative, 225
exons, 48
exposure, xii, xiii, 8, 9, 10, 23, 30, 74, 79, 81, 110, 112, 121, 126, 127, 171, 173, 185, 193, 215
extracellular matrix, 5, 14, 49, 60, 63, 66
extracts, 131
extravasation, 191

F

families, 80
family members, 114
fat, 173, 175, 178, 180, 181, 189, 195
fear, 114, 120
female rat, 74, 219
fibers, 49, 140
fibroblast growth factor, 32, 113, 123
fibrosis, 75, 83, 85, 180, 189, 195
filament, xi, 39, 50, 62
filters, 157
filtration, 178
fistulas, 75
fixation, 231, 235, 240
flight, 206
fluid, 92
fluorescence, 203, 211
Ford, 250
formation, x, 2, 4, 8, 18, 20, 22, 23, 34, 41, 43, 50, 68, 73, 100, 126, 127, 128, 133, 156, 172, 207, 215
fragility, 117

fragments, 94, 134
France, 82, 149, 225
free radicals, 73
freezing, 204
functional analysis, 67
fusion, 67

G

GE, 225
gel, 132, 205, 206
gene, 215, 216, 224, 226
gene amplification, 34, 48
gene expression, x, 2, 9, 42, 51, 53, 55, 77, 81, 226
gene therapy, 224
general anaesthesia, 118
general anesthesia, 142
genes, ix, x, 2, 5, 6, 7, 20, 23, 25, 26, 27, 40, 46, 47, 51, 53, 61, 66, 67, 69, 78, 80, 88, 135, 215, 225
genetic alteration, 7, 9, 11, 19, 40, 46
genetic mutations, 9
genetics, 30
genome, 4, 23
genomics, 200, 204
germ line, 6
Germany, 242
gingival, xi, 17, 31, 32, 40
gingival epithelium, 17, 31
gland, 4, 14, 15, 127, 135
glottis, 230, 231, 246, 248
glucose, 183, 196
glutathione, 88
glycoproteins, 25, 51
google, xiv, 149
grading, 86
grants, 134
granules, 100
granulomas, 105
groups, xv, xvi, 214, 215, 219, 220, 222, 223
guidance, 142
guidelines, 195

H

hair, 92, 99, 105
half-life, 79
HE, 30, 65, 70, 216
head, 214, 215, 223, 224, 225, 226, 227
head and neck cancer, xi, 11, 30, 32, 36, 63, 65, 66, 69, 71, 72, 81, 83, 87, 210, 211, 214, 215, 223, 225, 226, 227
healing, 114
health, 77
hemoglobin, 247
heterogeneity, 12, 13
high risk, 214
histological examination, 201
histology, xv, 22, 82, 200
history, 15, 111, 112, 117
homes, 114
Hong Kong, 106
host, 28, 215
Hungary, 242
Hunter, 46, 66
hybrid, 92
hybridization, 63, 67, 107
hydrogen, 218
hydrogen peroxide, 218
hypermethylation, 47, 54, 79, 200, 204, 209, 211
hyperplasia, 20, 22, 41, 43, 79, 101
hypersensitivity, 173, 193
hypothesis, 3, 6, 7, 8, 35, 83, 89, 192, 224
hypoxia, 27
hypoxia-inducible factor, 27

I

ideal, xv, 200
identification, ix, 1, 12, 13, 77, 131, 207, 208, 210
identity, 55
idiopathic, 22
IL-8, 211
imbalances, 63
immune function, 26

immune regulation, 126
immune response, 28
immunoglobulin, 5
immunohistochemical, 226
immunohistochemistry, 223
immunoreactivity, 50, 62, 68, 80, 81, 102
immunosuppression, 73
immunosurveillance, 3
impacted teeth, 217
improvements, 157
in situ hybridization, xii, 91, 93, 94, 107, 211
in vitro, 18, 30, 31, 134, 136, 137
in vivo, 31, 32, 53, 89
inactivation, 215
incidence, 33, 72, 74, 75, 77, 81, 82, 113, 127, 140, 214, 215, 224, 225, 226, 243
incisors, 33
incubation, 218
India, 72, 73
individuals, 173, 193, 202, 203, 205, 206, 208
inducer, 26, 80
induction, xiii, 29, 73, 78, 79, 126, 192, 196, 215, 232, 247
induction chemotherapy, 192, 196, 232, 247
induration, 75
infection, xii, 14, 83, 91, 101, 102, 151
inflammation, 14, 94, 95, 151, 182
infrastructure, 208
infundibulum, 100
ingestion, 151
inguinal, 103
inhibition, 33, 36, 37, 52, 53, 58, 79, 88, 136, 215
inhibitor, 7, 79, 80, 132, 133
inhomogeneity, 173
initiation, 3, 7, 8, 19, 26, 29, 31, 47
injury, 19, 28, 77, 133, 194, 201, 248
insults, 215
integration, x, 2, 28, 29, 81, 215
integrin, 51, 63
integrity, 56
intensity, 219, 220, 223
interface, 45, 182, 186

interferon, 113
intervention, xiii, 140, 160
intracranial aneurysm, 194
intravenously, 30
invasive, 215
invasive cancer, 20, 41
iodinated contrast, 161, 166, 173
iodinated contrast material, 161, 166
iodine, 166
ionization, 206
ionizing radiation, 79, 172, 173, 180, 185, 193
ipsilateral, 76, 171, 178
iron, 73
irradiation, xiii, 126, 127, 128, 129, 132, 133, 151, 239, 244, 245, 246, 248
Islam, 84
islands, 49, 80
isolation, 33
isopentane, 217
issues, xv, 200
Italy, 85, 91, 155, 241, 242

J

Japan, 134, 139, 142, 144
Jordan, 11, 32, 81, 201, 209, 211

K

keratin, xi, 17, 20, 22, 39, 43, 44, 45, 49, 50, 56, 61, 62, 94, 95, 150, 152
keratinocyte, xi, 23, 33, 40, 81
keratinocytes, xi, 17, 40, 113
keratosis, 100
kidney, 66, 194
kill, 79
killer cells, 113
kinases, 215
kinetics, xi, 72

L

labeling, 80
laminin-5, 113
laryngeal cancer, 231, 244, 245, 249
laryngectomy, 232, 233, 234, 235, 236, 241, 242, 243, 244, 245, 247, 249, 250
laryngoscopy, 230, 234
larynx, xvi, 72, 141, 157, 182, 229, 230, 231, 232, 233, 234, 235, 236, 239, 240, 241, 242, 244, 245, 246, 247, 248, 249, 250
latency, 102
Latin America, 72
lead, x, 2, 6, 9, 18, 118, 141, 146, 172
lesions, x, xiv, xv, 2, 10, 11, 18, 24, 40, 43, 45, 46, 48, 49, 68, 74, 75, 77, 78, 79, 80, 81, 84, 93, 96, 100, 101, 107, 114, 149, 186, 192, 200, 201, 202, 209, 210, 215, 216, 226, 233, 234, 235, 236, 242
leukemia, ix, xv, 2, 5, 18, 32, 35, 134, 200
leukoplakia, xi, 24, 71, 74, 84, 85, 201, 209, 210, 226
levator, xii, 92, 98
lichen, 75, 85, 211
lichen planus, 75, 85, 211
lifetime, 49
ligand, 4, 26, 48, 65, 134, 135
light, 63, 203
liquid chromatography, 209
liquid nitrogen, 217, 218
localization, 26, 51, 54, 57, 62, 134, 173
loci, 29, 41, 65
low risk, 102, 110
lower lip, 73, 75, 76, 84
lumen, 94, 166, 171
lung cancer, 10, 11, 25, 28, 30, 31, 34, 40, 43, 45, 52, 63, 64, 65, 66, 67, 68, 69, 70, 120
lysis, xiv, 113, 149

M

machinery, x, 2

macromolecules, 9
macrophages, 44
magnetic field, 172, 173, 182
magnetic moment, 172
magnetic resonance, 117, 195, 196, 230
magnetic resonance imaging, 117, 195, 230
magnetization, 173, 178
majority, 5, 6, 62, 110, 112, 232, 234
mammalian cells, 127
mammals, 26, 80
man, xii, 91, 93, 101, 143
management, 77, 114, 123, 194, 211, 245, 247, 248, 249
mandible, 141, 153
manipulation, 141
mapping, 64
mass, xii, 24, 49, 92, 93, 102, 120, 166, 200, 205, 206, 212
mass spectrometry, 200, 205, 206, 212
materials, 157, 216
matrix, 35, 45, 92, 99, 105, 113, 123, 126, 135
matrix metalloproteinase, 35, 113, 123
maxillary sinus, 123, 189
media, 173
median, 112, 145, 223
medical, xvi, 93, 114, 150, 229, 235
medical reason, 235
medicine, 3
medulloblastoma, 7, 27
melanoma, 27, 28, 30, 32, 33, 72, 79, 104
meninges, 166
mesenchyme, 52
mesothelioma, 67
messenger RNA, 65
meta-analysis, 107
metabolic changes, 201
metabolism, 26, 73, 83, 183, 192, 196
metabolites, 41
metabolized, 8, 183
metabolizing, 8
metalloproteinase, 64
metaphor, 3
metastases, 224, 227

metastasis, xi, xiv, 3, 5, 18, 33, 34, 35, 60, 67, 69, 71, 76, 77, 78, 85, 87, 103, 119, 140, 141, 146, 147, 150, 151, 152
metastatic cancer, 18, 20, 41
metastatic disease, 9, 120, 121, 183, 193
methodology, 224
methylation, 42, 200, 204
mice, 4, 15, 19, 31, 113
microcirculation, 180, 190, 191, 193
micronutrients, 83
microRNA, 204, 210
migration, 114, 115, 116, 231
Ministry of Education, 134
Minneapolis, 199
mitochondria, 49, 80
mitogen, 33
mitosis, 79, 81, 126, 129, 136, 152
mixing, 143, 144
models, 7, 15, 57, 197
mole, 114
molecular biology, 225
molecular weight, xi, 39, 62, 129, 130, 132
molecules, 3, 17, 32, 48, 56, 60, 67, 205, 208
monoclonal, 218
monoclonal antibody, 120, 218
morbidity, 118
morphogenesis, 66
morphology, xiv, 22, 155, 160
mortality, 82
Moscow, 28, 30, 36, 37
mouse, 218
mouth, 217, 226
MRI, xiii, xiv, 117, 140, 142, 155, 156, 171, 172, 173, 175, 180, 182, 186, 189, 193, 195, 196, 230
mRNA, 204, 211
mucosa, xv, 10, 11, 23, 24, 33, 47, 49, 62, 72, 78, 79, 80, 81, 84, 89, 99, 118, 158, 171, 214, 215, 216, 219, 220, 221, 222, 224, 226, 227, 231
multiples, 127
muscles, xii, 92, 166, 231
mycosis fungoides, 100
myosin, 206

N

nasopharyngeal carcinoma, 194
nasopharynx, 80
natural killer cell, 113
neck, 214, 215, 223, 224, 225, 226, 227
neck cancer, 65, 195, 196, 215, 223, 225,
    226, 227
necrosis, 43, 45, 121, 164, 166, 173
neoangiogenesis, 192
neoplasm, 50, 72, 80, 100, 152, 166, 173,
    178
neoplastic, 225
neoplastic tissue, 36, 225
neovascularization, 3
Nepal, 139
nephropathy, 194
nerve, 118
neuroendocrine cells, 22
nevus, 100
New England, 209
New South Wales, 109
nitric oxide, 88
nitric oxide synthase, 88
nitrogen, 217, 218
nodes, xvi, 76, 115, 152, 186, 189, 190, 229,
    230, 234, 235
nodules, 114, 117
nonsense mutation, 113
normal, xv, 214, 215, 216, 218, 224, 225
nuclear, 218
nuclear membrane, 80
nuclei, 43, 44, 49, 50, 78, 131, 132, 133,
    135, 219
nucleotide sequence, 4
nucleus, xiii, 4, 25, 44, 49, 58, 60, 126, 129,
    134, 136
nutrition, 73

O

odontogenic, 225
oesophageal, 115
oil, 29

omission, 218
oncogene, 218, 227
oncogenes, 3, 4, 5, 7, 47, 69, 225
oncogenesis, xi, 27, 31, 71, 89
oncology, 227
opportunities, 34
organ, x, 2, 13, 14, 33, 87, 101, 107, 166,
    182, 197, 244
organelles, 126
organism, x, 2, 9
organize, x, 2
organs, ix, x, 2, 39, 40, 62, 102, 156, 157,
    166, 171, 207
ovarian cancer, xv, 27, 34, 200
oxygen, 192

P

p21WAF1/CIP1, 88
p53, xv, xvi, 7, 11, 20, 26, 27, 29, 33, 46,
    47, 51, 68, 70, 78, 79, 88, 214, 215, 216,
    218, 219, 220, 222, 223, 224, 225, 226,
    227
paclitaxel, 87
pain, xiv, xv, 75, 114, 149, 151, 200
palate, 24, 50, 72, 74, 75, 115, 151, 164,
    167
palliative, 120
paper, 216
paradigm shift, 37
parallel, x, 2, 49, 157, 160, 196
parenchyma, 21
pathogenesis, 11, 27, 33, 37, 79, 92, 102,
    110, 112, 215
pathology, xii, 30, 82, 91, 92, 102
pathways, x, 2, 9, 12, 24, 32, 33, 36, 51, 64,
    79, 224
patients, xv, xvi, 214, 215, 216, 219, 220,
    223, 224, 225, 226, 227
pelvis, 98, 117
peptide, 205, 206, 212
peptides, 205, 206
perforation, 76
perfusion, xiv, 156, 180, 190, 191, 192, 193,
    195, 196, 197

periodontal, 151
permeability, 192
permission, iv
peroxide, 218
PET, xiv, 117, 155, 183, 185, 186, 193, 194, 195, 230
PET scan, 118
pharynx, 72, 82, 157, 226
phenotype, 5, 12, 31, 33, 36, 53, 86, 88, 113
phenotypes, x, 2, 19
Philadelphia, 244, 247
phosphate, 93, 218
phosphorylation, 52, 58, 127
photographs, 114
photons, 172
physical inactivity, 73
physical interaction, 113
physics, 193
pilot study, 196
plaque, 74, 123
plasma cells, 44
plasma membrane, 126
plastic surgeon, 117
platform, 25, 205, 211
play, xv, 214, 215, 223
pleura, 67
plexus, 230
pneumonia, 63
polarity, 56
pollutants, 41
polymerase, xii, 91, 93, 101
polymerase chain reaction, xii, 91, 93, 101
polypeptides, xi, 39
pons, 149
pools, 15
population, 5, 12, 13, 14, 17, 18, 19, 22, 31, 72, 74, 85, 110, 202, 214, 225, 226
positive correlation, 224
positron, 117, 196
positron emission tomography, 117, 196
precancer, 73, 81, 211
precipitation, 113
precursor cells, 5, 40, 43
preparation, iv, 133, 244
preservation, 197, 232, 233, 236, 244, 246

prevention, 65, 114, 115, 210, 224
primary tumor, xvi, 3, 6, 10, 11, 18, 19, 77, 140, 157, 185, 214, 215, 223, 224, 227, 229, 234
principles, 34
probability, 8, 18, 224
probe, 142, 143
producers, 73
professionals, 114
progenitor cells, 14, 19, 23, 33, 36, 62
prognosis, xi, xiv, 40, 50, 57, 59, 60, 65, 68, 71, 76, 77, 78, 86, 88, 101, 118, 126, 146, 150, 152, 155, 202, 215
proliferation, ix, xi, 4, 6, 7, 8, 9, 13, 18, 25, 29, 32, 36, 53, 55, 59, 60, 65, 69, 71, 78, 88, 97, 100, 101, 104, 113, 127, 129, 226, 227
promoter, 5, 8, 9, 47, 88, 209, 211
propagation, 19
prostate cancer, 27, 29, 30, 35
prostate carcinoma, 29
protein, 218, 223, 225
proteins, x, xiii, 2, 3, 25, 39, 49, 50, 57, 60, 62, 80, 88, 126, 128, 129, 130, 131, 133, 134, 135, 136, 205, 206, 209, 212, 215, 218, 224
proteome, 209
proteomics, 200, 205, 206, 207, 209
protons, 172
proto-oncogene, 4, 5, 6, 63, 64, 80
prototypes, 101
pulp, 17, 31
purification, 134
pyogenic, 100, 105

Q

quality of life, 120
quantification, 190, 227

R

race, 84

radiation, xv, 73, 77, 79, 83, 117, 120, 145, 151, 156, 171, 172, 180, 183, 192, 196, 232, 233, 244, 245, 247, 248
Radiation, 229, 244, 245, 247, 248
radiation therapy, xv, 77, 156, 192, 232, 233, 244, 247
radiography, 230
radiotherapy, xiii, xvi, 77, 87, 103, 120, 121, 126, 141, 152, 195, 196, 227, 230, 239, 240, 241, 242, 243, 244, 245, 246, 247, 248, 249
reactive oxygen, 83
reading, 160
reagents, 204
real time, xiii, 140, 142, 145
receptors, 3, 4, 9, 25, 26, 27, 30, 54
recognition, 65
recommendations, iv
reconstruction, 119, 152, 158, 164, 166, 247
recovery, 17, 250
rectum, xii, 92
recurrence, xiv, 10, 35, 77, 103, 118, 119, 141, 146, 156, 180, 185, 189, 249
redistribution, 132
regeneration, 16, 17, 34
registries, 226
registry, 109, 122
regression, 29, 120
rehabilitation, 244
relaxation, 172
relevance, 86
reliability, 142, 208
repair, 9, 78, 215
replication, 78
repressor, 26
reproduction, 161
researchers, 3, 8, 27
resection, xiii, 119, 140, 141, 143, 146, 147, 152, 227, 245, 246, 248
residual disease, 236
resistance, 69, 126
resolution, xiv, 70, 142, 145, 156, 157, 160, 173, 180, 182, 192, 195, 196
respiratory, 226

response, 25, 27, 44, 48, 191, 192, 193, 196, 197, 225, 248
reticulum, 17, 80
retinoblastoma, 6, 48, 68, 78, 88
retroviruses, 4
risk, xii, xiii, 8, 9, 10, 12, 24, 46, 49, 50, 73, 74, 75, 77, 80, 81, 83, 91, 102, 110, 111, 112, 121, 122, 171, 194, 201, 214, 217, 224, 232, 233, 235, 243
risk factors, 46, 73, 74, 81, 217
risks, 82, 201
room temperature, 218
root, 105
routes, 208
rules, 165

S

S phase, 215
safety, xiv, 140, 141, 142, 143, 144, 145
saline, 217, 218
saliva, xv, 200, 203, 204, 205, 206, 208, 210, 211, 212
salivary gland, xiii, 27, 32, 135, 140, 186
salivary glands, 32
saturation, 178
Saudi Arabia, 213
science, 8, 204
secretion, 14, 152
seed, 3
seeding, 33
senescence, 47
sensitivity, 182, 186, 200, 202, 203, 204, 205, 206, 207
sepsis, xiii, 121
serine, 25
serum, 218
sex, 63, 84, 93, 145
sex ratio, 145
sexual contact, 102
shape, 142, 143, 144
showing, 56, 74, 76, 77, 100, 105, 117, 165, 167, 178, 205, 217, 220, 221, 222
side effects, 117
signal transduction, 4, 23, 25, 34, 51

signaling pathway, x, xi, 2, 4, 5, 24, 27, 35, 40, 52
signals, 3, 4, 25, 26, 27, 47
signal-to-noise ratio, 157
signs, 217
silver, 136
Singapore, 106
sinuses, 150, 151, 157
skeleton, 62, 66
skin, ix, xiii, 7, 8, 25, 29, 30, 31, 34, 57, 60, 108, 112, 113, 114, 115, 116, 117, 119, 120, 121, 122, 123, 124, 178, 234
skin cancer, 34, 115, 123
Slovenia, 226
smoking, 10, 28, 46, 63, 65, 67, 68, 84, 224, 226
smooth muscle, 70
smooth muscle cells, 70
software, 156
solid tumors, 18, 32
solidification, 143, 144
solution, 142, 144, 203
South Africa, 84, 239
Southeast Asia, 73
Spain, 1, 28, 39, 62
species, 8, 9, 15, 36, 83
specifications, 15
speech, 75, 141
spin, 172, 194, 195
sputum, 67
stability, 54, 55, 62, 128, 136
stabilization, 80, 204
stars, 95
state, ix, xv, 2, 14, 31, 77, 113, 191, 200, 202
states, 18, 35
statistics, 68, 81, 82, 193, 244
stem cells, ix, x, 1, 2, 11, 12, 14, 15, 16, 17, 18, 19, 23, 28, 29, 30, 31, 32, 33, 34, 104
stenosis, 194
sternocleidomastoid, 178, 181, 182
stimulant, 113
stimulus, 7
stochastic model, 18
stoma, 234

stomach, xv, 200
storage, 217
stress, 47, 112, 122
stroke, 191
stroma, 60
stromal cells, 53
structure, 4, 7, 15, 55, 56, 65, 101, 134
subcutaneous tissue, 178
subdomains, 56
substrate, 134, 218
suicide, 135
sulfate, 60
Sun, 27, 35
superimposition, 131
support staff, 244
suppression, 37, 173, 178, 194, 195
suppressor, 215, 225
Surgery, 213
surgical intervention, 120
surgical resection, 141, 185
survival, x, xv, 2, 19, 27, 31, 35, 60, 69, 76, 77, 81, 82, 85, 141, 150, 151, 200, 202, 208, 215, 224, 225, 232, 236, 243
susceptibility, 7, 80, 123, 182
Sweden, 72, 83, 209
symptoms, 74, 75
synchronous, 223
syndrome, 73, 100, 104, 105
synthesis, 113
systems, 226

T

T cell, 28, 29, 55
Taiwan, 74, 226
tar, 31, 35
target, 9, 25, 27, 33, 51, 54, 55, 79, 136, 137, 191
targeted drug development, 210
techniques, xiv, 155, 189, 192, 193, 194, 195, 224
technologies, xv, 200, 204, 208
technology, xiv, 156, 157
teeth, 36, 75, 151, 217
temperature, 218

tendon, 117
tendons, 118
tension, 192
terminal patients, 75
territory, 161
testing, 201, 202, 203, 208
TGF, 27, 36, 48
Thailand, 86
theory, 215
therapeutic change, 195
therapeutic targets, xiii, 89, 121
therapy, xiv, 10, 30, 79, 87, 124, 134, 141,
    150, 152, 185, 189, 192, 197, 214, 224,
    247, 248, 249
three-dimensional reconstruction, 107
threonine, 25
thyroid, 80, 165, 171, 173, 230, 231, 234,
    235
time, 215
tissue, ix, x, xii, xiii, 1, 2, 3, 5, 8, 9, 10, 13,
    14, 17, 19, 26, 34, 44, 45, 62, 65, 76, 91,
    92, 93, 112, 113, 118, 140, 142, 158,
    161, 164, 166, 171, 172, 183, 189, 190,
    191, 195, 202, 203, 204, 215, 216, 217,
    218, 224, 236, 248
TNF, 211
tobacco, 41, 46, 70, 73, 74, 201, 209, 215,
    219, 220, 224
tobacco smoke, 41, 73
tobacco smoking, 224
tooth, 17, 36
toxicity, 120
trachea, 15, 19, 231
tracheostomy, 232, 234
transcription, x, 2, 4, 25, 27, 51, 53, 55, 58
transcription factors, x, 2, 4, 25, 51, 55
transcripts, 204
transduction, x, 2
transferrin, 206, 210
transformation, ix, xi, xii, 2, 5, 9, 10, 15, 17,
    23, 32, 43, 45, 49, 66, 71, 73, 75, 79, 81,
    85, 92, 99, 100, 104, 201, 211
transforming growth factor, 27, 65
transgene, 32
transition, 215

translocation, 5, 80, 89
transmembrane glycoprotein, 56
transmission, 4, 83
transplant, 84
transplantation, 101, 107
trauma, ix, xiii, 2, 84, 112, 121, 151
trial, 87, 117, 123, 247
triggers, 9
turnover, xi, 40, 126
tyrosine, xiii, 48, 51, 121

U

ulcer, 24, 49, 106, 114
ultrasonography, 140, 147
ultrasound, 117, 145, 147, 186
unmasking, 224
urinary bladder, ix, 80
users, 220

V

validation, 207, 208
variables, 77, 216, 219
variations, 100
vegetables, 73
vein, 164
ventricle, 230
viral, 215
viral infection, 201
viruses, 4
visualization, 114
vitamins, 73

W

war, 215
Washington, 64, 237, 241, 242
water, 166, 173, 175, 180, 182
Western blot, xiii, 126, 129, 130, 132, 206
World Health Organization (WHO), 76, 82,
    226
windows, 158

Wisconsin, 242
WM, 226
Wnt signaling, xi, 25, 29, 35, 36, 40, 51, 53, 55, 68, 70
workers, 77
worldwide, xv, 72, 82, 200, 214

Y

yield, 191
young people, 84